DIET STACKING™

FIND YOUR STACK
AND LOSE WEIGHT FAST!

DAWNA STONE

First Edition: May 2019

ISBN 978-0-9992123-5-6

Cover design and formatting by Archangel Ink.

Healthy You Ventures, LLC

CONTENTS

LET'S DO IT TOGETER!

TAKE THE ONLINE DIET STACKING WEIGHT LOSS CHALLENGE!

Stacking Videos…Beginner's Guide…
Meal Plans…Shopping Lists…Diet Stacking
Rules…50+ Recipes (with photos)…Diet
Stacking Approved Diets…FAQ's…and more!

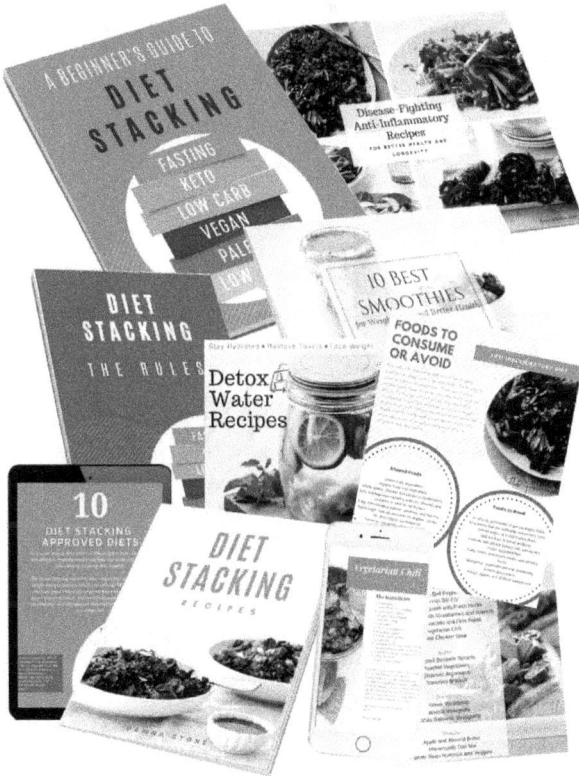

LEARN MORE AND SIGN UP AT
DAWNASTONE.COM/DIETSTACKING

INTRODUCTION:
IT'S TIME TO STACK!

Michele stayed on the Keto diet for nearly a month and lost over 10 pounds. Although she saw great results, she couldn't find the motivation to stay on the diet any longer. She got tired of eating so few carbohydrates and struggled to get the recommended fat intake. She knew the diet had scientifically-proven health benefits, but those insights just weren't enough to keep her on the diet. As she stopped following the program, she slowly reverted back to her old habits, and within 60 days, she had gained back all the weight she had worked so hard to lose.

Sarah researched the Paleo diet and decided to give it a try. The first day went smoothly, and she thought she was finally on her way to losing those unwanted pounds. But mid-way through day three, she struggled to stick to the plan. By day four she gave in and returned to her old eating habits. She felt as though she failed yet again and decided Paleo just wasn't for her. She vowed to not give up on her weight loss goals but to find a diet that's right for her. She's still searching.

Joe and his wife found success with the Atkins diet. They even touted their low-carb lifestyle to friends and family. Each lost over 20 pounds and felt great. The diet however wasn't sustainable. Their social lifestyle made adhering to the program difficult. And as the struggle became more and more difficult, they gave up on their low-carb lifestyle all together. When they went back to their previous ways of eating, the weight piled back on. Both felt the diet wasn't a good long-term solution.

The Keto diet, the Paleo diet, and the Atkins diet have all been proven to work as have many other top-rated diets. The Mediterranean diet, intermittent fasting, and the anti-inflammatory diet are some others that deserve mention. And all have many scientifically-proven health benefits that you will read about in the chapters to follow. The problem, however, is that most people find these diets difficult to "stick to" for long periods of time, and as their motivation wanes (or diminishes all together), so does their ability to follow the plan.

If you can relate to any of these stories, you're not alone. So many of us start a diet fully committed and motivated to finally succeed. Unfortunately, it's human nature to lose motivation over time. What may seem exciting and very doable on day one can often feel impossible by day four. This is where Diet Stacking comes to the rescue! Diet Stacking provides a structure that allows you to keep your motivation high over a much longer period of time—allowing for greater success and sustained weight loss.

So what is Diet Stacking? Diet Stacking is the process of stacking one diet on top of another as a way to maintain a high level of motivation and willpower. Research shows that motivation diminishes over time, and peak motivation only lasts for a few days before diminishing. 95% of weight loss attempts fail. Why? They fail because people lose their motivation and no longer feel they can stay within the limits of the diets they have chosen.

Diet Stacking is the silver bullet in the quest to find a long-term solution to weight loss. Diet Stacking allows for a continued burst of motivation (motivation that often fades when a single diet is used alone). By stacking the best scientifically proven weight loss diets, you can reap the rewards of each diet—weight loss, better health, disease prevention, and more—without the motivational struggle to adhere to the same strict dietary rules for weeks, months or years. Want a program that is specifically designed to help you not only lose weight but keep it off for the long term? Diet Stacking is for you!

The average person goes through the following eight stages when starting a new diet or weight loss plan:

Stage One: Decision-Making

In stage one, we decide that we need to eat better or lose weight. Once that decision is made, we move on to stage two.

Stage Two: Planning

In this stage, we start planning how we are going to achieve our weight loss goals. During this stage, we typically choose our specific diet program or start setting diet rules for ourselves.

Stage Three: Determining Timing

In stage three, we set a start date (often a Monday) and determine how long we are willing to commit to our new diet (often a 7, 10, 15, 21 or 30-day time period).

Stage Four: Building Excitement

With our plan and start date set, we get excited about the success that we believe will come from finally achieving our goals.

Stage Five: Motivation Peaks

Stage five directly aligns with the first day of our new diet. This is the day that we've been waiting for. Our motivation is off the charts, and we feel exhilarated about our decision to make positive changes in our eating and lifestyle.

Stage Six: Motivation Tapers Off

In stage six, we remain motivated to reap the reward of our diet, but the initial excitement has lessened. We slowly begin to realize that our new diet is going to take some serious effort on our part to succeed in reaching our goals.

Stage Seven: Motivation Erodes Further

In stage seven, we try to find the mental toughness to continue, but we gradually start to wonder, "Is the effort really worth it?"

Stage Eight: Motivation is Replaced with Defeat

In this final stage, we have completely given up on our weight loss goals and blame ourselves for a lack of willpower.

We give up and resort back to our old ways. We might even binge or go to opposite dietary extremes for a few days.

With Diet Stacking, you can avoid the classic "Eight-Stage" experience that most have when dieting. Diet Stacking is your key to finding the motivation and willpower to succeed in achieving your weight loss goals. With Diet Stacking, you get a surge of new inspiration and excitement just before you start losing motivation. By stacking different diets, you stay just as excited throughout your diet plan as you were when you decided to take that first step! Just when most people are getting ready to throw in the towel, you enjoy a boost in motivation and excitement over and over again. That is what Diet Stacking can do for you!

By choosing to Diet Stack, you avoid the majority of the unwanted stages of dieting. Just as you start to feel hopeless in stage seven when your motivation begins to wane, you jump right back into stage four and become reenergized about the new diet that will start the following day. And instead of entering stage eight and feeling like a failure, you repeatedly gain a sense of empowerment as your motivation is reinvigorated. With Diet Stacking, you make the switch at the perfect time so that your chances of weight-loss success are the greatest.

Diet Stacking disrupts the normal dieting process and allows you to experience enhanced motivation and more willpower over the long term. Diet Stacking turns typical dieting on its head by eliminating the number one reason people fail to stick to a diet and lose weight—diminishing willpower and motivation. Diet Stacking is the secret to staying motivated and reaching your weight loss goals! Sound appealing? Then keep reading to find out how Diet Stacking can work for you!

Download your **free Beginner's Guide to Diet Stacking** for quick and easy access to the art of Stacking. Download now: https://dawnastone.com/beginners-guide-to-diet-stacking

JOIN ME FOR THE DIET STACKING WEIGHT LOSS CHALLENGE!

Want to Stack together? Sign up for the online Diet Stacking challenge. As part of the program, you will receive:

Four video tutorials

- Welcome video
- The Simple Stack explained
- The Weight Loss Stack explained
- The Extreme Stack explained

Detailed and easy-to-follow meal plans

- Simple Stack Meal Plan
- Weight Loss Stack Meal Plan
- Extreme Stack Meal Plan

Shopping lists

50+ Diet Stacking Recipes (with photos)

Frequently Asked Questions Handbook

In addition, you will receive **three downloadable guides** to help ensure your success:

- The Beginner's Guide to Diet Stacking
- Diet Stacking Success Tips
- Diet Stacking 101: The Rules

Plus, if you sign up today, you'll receive **three incredible bonuses**!

- 4 Anti-Inflammatory Recipes
- 27 Detox Water Recipes
- 10 Best Smoothies

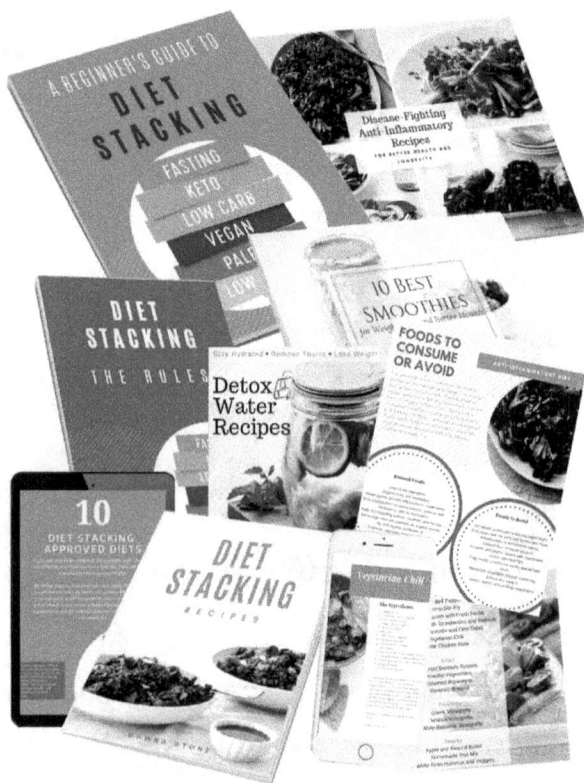

Find out more and sign up at
DawnaStone.com/DietStacking

SECTION I:

DIET STACKING 101

CHAPTER 1:

WHY WEIGHT LOSS IS SO DIFFICULT

At some point in time, most of us have gone on a diet. Our incentive might have been to simply be healthier or to have more energy throughout the day. But most choose to diet in an effort to lose excess weight. No matter the reason, most of the time our ability to achieve (and sustain) our goals falls short. For one reason or another, we start out strong only to lose momentum as time passes. And before long, we are right back where we started…or in some cases, even farther from our goals.

Several research studies have shown that our ability to succeed in dieting pursuits is severely lacking. In fact, researchers from the University of Minnesota and UCLA reviewed dozens of studies related to dieting and long-term weight loss. What they found was rather disheartening. While most people on diets did lose weight the first several months, almost all had gained the weight back, plus a couple of extra pounds, two to five years later.[1] Thus, it is understandable why skepticism abounds when it comes to new dieting strategies.

Unfortunately, we are in the midst of a major global epidemic when it comes to being overweight or obese. According to the Centers for Disease Control and Prevention, nearly 40 percent of all Americans are obese, and more than half are overweight. Similar statistics are now being reported worldwide. And, notably, obesity is linked to many poor health outcomes. Heart disease, diabetes, stroke, and high blood pressure are just a few of the more serious ones.[2] It stands to reason that paying greater attention to our diets is needed perhaps more than ever.

This is where Diet Stacking offers hope. Diet Stacking is a revolutionary concept that can help you lose the weight you want and keep it off. Specifically, Diet Stacking addresses some of the most common obstacles that prevent you from achieving your weight loss goals while honoring healthy eating habits and proper nutrition. The more we learn about how our bodies react to dieting, and the more we understand about human motivation, the better we are in our approach to healthy weight loss. Diet Stacking considers these new insights and offers you a better way!

Looking Back at Dieting Approaches Over Time

Dieting is certainly not a novel idea. In fact, the word diet comes from the ancient Greek word "diaita," which refers to eating specific foods for the purpose of weight loss and better health. The Greeks adopted some healthy approaches to dieting, but they also had some that were clearly not so healthy. Daily purging when overweight is one example of a less than desirable weight loss approach. Regardless, the association between diet, weight loss and health has been appreciated for a long time.

While dieting was prominent during the ancient Greek and Roman cultures, it really took off after the 18th century.

Rich foods and rising wealth meant upper-class members of society were packing on the pounds. Ultimately, this caused dieting to become more popular. In the 1800s, high protein, low carb diet fads gained momentum. And by the early 20th century, celebrity endorsements were in vogue.[3] It's a small leap to see where these trends have taken us today.

It seems like there are an infinite number of diet plans on the market today, each with its own unique advantages and disadvantages. But despite this, we are hardly better off when it comes to controlling our weight. How can this be? While some of the answers lie in how our bodies respond to a particular diet, others simply involve human nature. Understanding how both of these factors play a role in dieting is important when considering innovative approaches to healthy weight loss.

Old Science Versus New Science

For many who have dieted over the years, one common formula may sound familiar. In order to lose one pound in weight, all you need to do is cut back your calorie intake by 3,500 calories. So, if you reduce your diet by 1,000 calories a day, assumedly you will lose a couple of pounds each week. This is known as the Wishofsky rule based on research done years ago. But there is only one problem…the formula isn't very accurate.

More recent research shows that our ability to lose weight by cutting back on our calories varies over time. In fact, there are two phases of weight loss whenever we start a diet. During the first few days to weeks, weight loss is more rapid. It seems to take a much smaller decrease in your calorie intake to shed the pounds. But unfortunately, this all changes in the second phase. After a week or so, your body's metabolism slows in response to your diet change. From then on, you have to cut back even further on your calories to see the same response.[4]

How many times have you started a diet and seen great results in that first week? If you are trying to lose weight for some big event, this can certainly work to your advantage. This can also serve as great feedback in motivating you to stick to your diet. But then the "slowdown" phase kicks in, and your weight loss seems to slow to a crawl. Based on what science has shown about dieting and your metabolism, it makes perfect sense. But that hardly gives you a strong incentive to keep going.

Motivation Is the Key to Dieting Success

As science has shown, weight loss still occurs with dieting over time, even though it is slower than desired. But most of us simply do not persevere. What obstacles are in the way to keep us from realizing our weight loss goals? Based on surveys of men and women, three barriers seem to be the most important…time, taste and motivation.[5] Naturally, time is a precious commodity today for all of us, and taste for specific foods is quite individualized. But all of us have the potential to improve our motivation, and this is where Diet Stacking can make a significant difference.

When it comes to motivation, a number of theories can help us identify how to best go about dieting. One of the most well known theories is Maslow's Hierarchy of Needs. In this motivational theory, various needs are ranked according to their level of priority. Physiological and safety needs, for example, are among the highest priorities. Certainly, having enough food is a basic need that motivates us to eat. Other needs are only considered after these basic needs are met, like the need for belonging and a positive sense of self-esteem. These are more likely to drive dieting and weight loss pursuits.

While Maslow's theory helps us understand our basic motivation to stick to a diet, it does not exactly explain why diets often fail. Another motivational theory provides greater insight in this regard. Vroom's Expectancy Theory of Motivation identifies three specific areas of motivation. These areas include the effort we put forth in dieting, whether or not we think the effort will produce results, and the actual value we assign to weight loss.[6] These appear to actually have more relevance when it comes to weight loss and dieting.

For many diets, the amount of effort it takes to stay on the diet undermines its value to us. As time passes, eating the same types of foods and restricting calories becomes more of a struggle. This naturally reduces our level of motivation over time. Likewise, as the weight loss slows, our belief that our efforts will produce the results we want fades. We still want to lose the weight, but our motivation becomes less and less because we're simply not convinced the struggle is worth it. Wouldn't it be nice if there was a diet that helped you overcome these challenges in your motivation?

Diet Stacking – A Fresh Look at Dieting

With an understanding of the realities of dieting, the challenges of successful weight loss become increasingly clear. First, while diets can help you achieve a healthier weight, their ability to be nutritious and meet your basic health needs is also essential. Second, healthy diets do not necessarily keep producing the same amount of weight loss over time…unfortunately. Appreciating this can at least help you know what to expect over time. Lastly, if we can maintain a higher level of motivation, the opportunity for success increases tremendously. Diet Stacking address all three of these "realities" when it comes to weight loss success.

In the next chapter, the concept and practice of Diet Stacking will be explained in greater detail. But without question, Diet Stacking can help you better achieve the weight loss results you want. Millions of people struggle with weight issues today, and a new approach is needed given the longstanding history of diet failures. By applying current evidence to better dieting practices, Diet Stacking provides a novel way to not only promote weight loss now but also help you maintain the weight you desire into the future.

CHAPTER 2:

WHY DIET STACKING WORKS

Having discussed the challenges involved with weight loss and dieting, you can appreciate why a new approach is needed. Many of the diets recommended today offer numerous benefits. In fact, several offer healthy ways to lose weight while providing nutritious meal plans. But even with these select diets, the ability to stick to the plan often fades over time. A lack of quick results and the effort involved slowly erodes our motivation. Before long, our best intentions to lose weight and be healthy give in to temptations to cut corners. And eventually, we find ourselves reverting back to our same old habits.

What's the solution to these challenges? Isn't there a way to diet over the long-haul while maintaining a focus on our weight loss and health goals? Yes, there is! Diet Stacking provides a new strategy that preserves the benefits of many healthy diet plans while boosting motivation and results. You may be less than optimistic that such a diet plan exists given all the diets you have tried. But rest assured, Diet Stacking is not like anything you have ever tried before.

The Eight Common Stages of Dieting

Before describing Diet Stacking in greater detail and its potential for healthy weight loss, it helps to revisit what most people experience when trying a new diet. From start to finish, eight common stages can usually be identified. And while some of the early stages will be the same for Diet Stacking, those that signal eminent failure can be better avoided.

Stage One: Decision Making

You may think about losing weight and eating a healthier diet often, but the actual dieting process doesn't begin until you decide to do something about it. Like any endeavor, dieting begins with a steadfast decision to take action.

Stage Two: Planning

Once the decision has been made to diet, you then determine how you want to go about it. This includes choosing your diet and knowing which dieting rules you will follow.

Stage Three: Determining Timing

With a plan in place, you now identify your weight loss and health goals, and you determine how long you will be on your diet plan and when you will start.

Stage Four: Building Excitement

With everything now in place, it's time to get started. Building excitement to launch your dieting plan might involve buying new foods, creating new schedules, and simply envisioning the weight you will lose.

Stage Five: Motivation Peaks

Usually on the first day of your diet, your levels of motivation and excitement are off the charts. You will feel empowered to succeed and committed to persevere.

Stage Six: Motivation Tapers Off

Though you are still motivated to achieve your weight loss goals, the initial excitement has faded and you appreciate the actual effort that will be involved. This often occurs around the second and third days of the diet.

Stage Seven: Motivation Erodes Further

Sticking to the diet begins to get tougher and tougher as you increasingly think about the foods you are missing. The positive feedback being received may not be enough to stay constantly focused on your weight loss goals. This may begin as early as the third day of the diet.

Stage Eight: Motivation is Replaced with Defeat

In this stage, you revert back to your old eating habits, and you might even binge. Realizing your lack of success in attaining your weight loss goals triggers feelings of defeat and self-blame. This can occur as early as the fourth day of your diet.

Do these eight stages of dieting sound familiar to you? If so, you are not alone. More than 95 percent of people attempting a diet fail to achieve their weight loss or health goals. And most diets fail within a week. As you can appreciate from the eight stages of dieting discussed, maintaining a high level of motivation is the biggest problem. And this is where Diet Stacking offers some of its most significant advantages.

What Is Diet Stacking?

Today, we live in an attention-deficit type of environment. Snippets of information bombard us all day long, and we now prefer to get our news in quick videos or soundbites. Regardless whether we think this is good or bad, it is a reality. And we have become accustomed to these types of interaction within our lives. Therefore, it makes logical sense that our ability to sustain attention for long periods of time has declined. In fact, a study performed by Microsoft® in 2015 showed than the average attention span fell from 12 seconds to 8 seconds over the course of the last 15 years.[7]

As human beings, we also crave variety. Mixing things up a bit keeps us engaged, interested, and involved. Research also supports this fact when looking at how to keep employees focused on their jobs. Jobs that allow people to use a variety of tasks and skills in their daily routine are naturally more engaged and productive. Compared to people who complete the same activities day after day, those who enjoy greater variety at work perform better over time.[8]

What do these research studies have to do with dieting? Actually, a lot! Think about the last time you went on a diet. Whatever diet you might have selected, there were rules that had to be followed. Rules meant you could include some foods in your diet plan and not others. It might have also meant having to eat very similar foods day after day. In retrospect, how did the lack of variety and rules affect your ability to stay on the diet? If you're like most people, the impact was probably pretty significant.

Keeping this in mind, Diet Stacking lets you combine a variety of different diets in a structured way to help you stay focused on your weight loss goals. Depending on which Diet Stacking plan or "stack" you choose, you cycle through several different diet programs over time. You participate in each diet in your stack for three days before moving onto the next one. In doing so, you get to sample a variety of different diets, all of which have been proven to be effective individually.

For example, suppose you choose a "simple stack" that consists of three specific diets. Your first diet might be an intermittent fasting (IF) diet. After you have been on the IF diet for three days, you might then switch to a ketogenic diet for the next three days. Finally, you complete your cycle with a vegan diet for three days. Through the process, you have "stacked" three diets together (or completed a "3-Stack") as part of your personalized Diet Stacking program. And once you have completed the cycle, you might then choose to start the process over again.

As will be described later in the book, the Diet Stack that you select may contain three, five or seven of the Diet Stacking approved diets. Alternatively, you may decide to customize your own Diet Stack using these diets. The primary benefit to this approach, other than the potential for sustained healthy weight loss, is Diet Stacking's ability to help you avoid boredom. Just when you are about to get tired of a specific meal plan or diet, it's time to switch to the next one! As you can see, Diet Stacking is perfect for those who prefer variety and shorter duration challenges.

As already mentioned, the different Diet Stacks are discussed in greater detail in chapters 14 through 18. But it makes sense to give you a high-level description of Diet Stacking before you move on to the Diet Stacking approved diets. Here are just a few high-level details to help you better understand the stacking process:

1) "Stacking" means completing one diet and then starting or "stacking" on your next diet.

2) Each diet in your Diet Stack only lasts for three days. After three days, you move on to the next diet in your stack.

3) There are infinite ways you can customize or personalize your Diet Stack. But the programs highlighted in the book—the Simple Stack, the Weight Loss Stack and the Extreme Stack—have been proven to work.

Diet Stacking—Overcoming Common Dieting Success Obstacles

By far, the biggest challenge for anyone dieting is staying motivated and having enough willpower to persevere. Many techniques can be used to increase motivation, and Diet Stacking takes advantage of several of them. In addition to variety, Diet Stacking boosts motivation by providing quick weight loss, adding excitement to your diet program, and reducing the amount of effort it takes to lose weight. The following details why Diet Stacking is a great new approach to healthy weight loss:

- *Cycling Through Your Diet Stack Is Fun!* – Every three days, you get to try a new diet in your approach to weight loss. In addition to avoiding the boredom that eventually sets in with a single diet program, Diet Stacking lets you sample a variety of diets three days at a time. This is naturally more fun and engaging. And the more engaged you are, the better your motivation and commitment will be!

- *Sticking to Your Diet Plan Takes Less Effort* – Motivation for any task is affected by the amount of effort you have to exert. Even if you value weight loss a great deal, a significant amount of effort to achieve your goals can affect your desire to keep going. With Diet Stacking, however, it takes less effort to diet. Why? Because the drudgery of having to eat the same meal plans and follow the same dietary rules for long periods of time is avoided! And less effort means you are more likely to stay on track.

- *Diet Stacking Increases Opportunities for Positive Feedback* – Most diets provide great incentives the first few days or weeks of the program as you lose several pounds. But in time, these positive results may be less and less profound. With Diet Stacking, you increase your chances for positive feedback during your dieting process. And even if your motivation starts to diminish after only a few days, you know you'll soon be changing to the next diet. Having the potential for more positive feedback as well as more control over the outcome and increased motivation naturally inspires you to continue with your plan.

- *The Potential for Greater Weight Loss Success* – If you consider other approaches to weight loss, like exercise, Diet Stacking may have additional benefits. Cross-training exercises boost metabolism by stimulating different energy systems in the body. It may be that Diet Stacking has similar effects through dietary "cross-training." The science of dieting and its effects on the body's hormone systems, metabolism, and brain reactions are still evolving. But the potential for Diet Stacking to offer some advantages here may very well exist also.

Diet Disruption—The Key Behind Diet Stacking

The choice to use the term "stacking" in the name Diet Stacking is an important one. In essence, you "stack" diets one after another in Diet Stacking no different than you would stack building blocks. One serves as a foundation for the next, and in the process, you achieve better results than you would using a single diet alone. The benefits of each diet can be realized, and potentially, the ultimate outcome is more than the sum of their parts. In this way, the stacking of diets offers a completely new strategy to weight loss.

But more importantly, the primary benefit of Diet Stacking relates to its "Diet Disruption." Single plan diets have repeatedly failed as numerous studies have shown. And the main reason they fail is due to a lack of motivation to persevere. By disrupting the dieting routine and schedule, Diet Stacking lets you have greater variety. This, in turn, helps boost motivation and interest. And the best part is that Diet Stacking offers a healthy approach to dieting success because it takes advantage of diets proven to be effective. In the next chapter, we will specifically describe which diets have been selected for the Diet Stacking program and the reasons behind this list of diets.

CHAPTER 3:

DIET STACKING APPROVED DIETS

As you are likely aware, dozens of diet programs exist. Some are very effective, and some offer benefits to specific individuals in specific situations. And still others are simply fads that come and go over time offering little long-term benefits. Understanding this as well as identifying which diets are the most effective and safest is important. Naturally, you don't want to waste your time on a diet that offers little chance of weight or health improvement. At the same time, you want diets that offer comprehensive wellness while also helping you lose weight.

In total, ten different diets can be considered when creating your own personalized Diet Stack. After careful consideration of dozens of diets currently used for weight loss, those selected reflect the ones that offer you the best potential for success. Current scientific research was reviewed to determine which diets offered the best opportunity to help you attain your ideal weight. In addition, the final selections recognized the fact that Diet Stacking involves the use of a particular diet for only 3 days at a time. Thus, the key criteria involved diets that offered weight loss relatively quickly, were easy to adopt and understand, and were identified as effective based on scientific evidence.

In addition to these considerations, the diets approved for Diet Stacking were also chosen based on their overall ability to promote health and wellness. While some diets may have great weight loss potential, they may not be the best option when it comes to your overall wellbeing. In these instances, your efforts can "backfire" on you. A diet may help you lose weight, but the way you feel over time undermines your ability to stick to the diet. Ultimately, this will result in an inability to achieve your long-term weight loss goals. Thus, the final decision regarding the Diet Stacking approved diets also included an assessment of their overall promotion of wellness.

An Overview of the Approved Diet Stacking Diets

The following descriptions of the ten Diet Stacking approved diets explain the rationale for their inclusion in the program. In later chapters, more in-depth details will be provided about each diet's specific approaches and best practices. I hope that this information will give you the insights that will help you decide which Diet Stacking approved diets are best for you. But presently, the following allows you to appreciate current evidence regarding each of the diets so that you will better understand each diet's potential and why each was selected as a Diet Stacking approved diet.

The Intermittent Fasting Diet

Remarkably, intermittent fasting has been shown to have tremendous health benefits in addition to weight loss advantages. Numerous reviews of the scientific literature support the intermittent fasting diet as highly effective for rapid weight loss. In one review, the range of weight loss include nearly 3 percent on one's body weight in a month up to 9 percent at 6 months.[9] Other studies show that your waistline also shrinks while on an intermittent fasting diet by as much a 7 percent.[10] And, people tend to stay on an intermittent fasting diet. Roughly 80 percent of people find it easy to stick to.[11]

Like the other diets selected for Diet Stacking, the intermittent fasting diet has notable health benefits in addition to effective weight loss potential. Research supports its effectiveness in reducing heart and vascular disease as well as reducing the risk for diabetes.[12] The intermittent fasting diet is also associated with reduced risks for some dementias and some cancers. And, the intermittent fasting diet allows you to keep your muscle mass while boosting your metabolism.[13] These great advantages of the intermittent fasting diet allow you to lose weight quickly while enhancing your overall well-being.

The Ketogenic Diet

Used initially to treat epilepsy, the ketogenic diet has been more recently recognized as being effective for weight loss. In research studies, the average weight loss among individuals on a ketogenic diet 3 months or more was 11 pounds.[14] And, the ketogenic diet specifically targets unwanted fatty tissue, especially located around the midline. Studies have shown that the average reduction in body mass index is 7 percent with selective loss of fat tissue percentages as high as 70 percent.[15] Not only does the ketogenic diet allow rapid weight loss in those areas you most want it, but it also does so while reducing your overall appetite and hunger levels.[16]

The ketogenic diet is simple to adopt once you appreciate the food options available to you. Also, the ketogenic diet has a number of secondary health effects beyond weight loss making it ideal for anyone trying to achieve wellness. Specifically, the ketogenic diet is associated with lower blood glucose levels, less insulin resistance, and lower triglycerides.[17] Many diabetics have actually been able to reverse diabetic problems on a ketogenic diet.[18] Given the available research concerning the ketogenic diet, its inclusion in the list of Diet Stacking approved diets is well supported.

The Low-Carb Diet

This Diet Stacking approved diet has plenty of research to back ups its merit as an effective and safe way to lose weight and is also easy to implement into your daily life. Numerous research studies have examined whether or not the low-carb diet is effective for weight loss. One study showed that the average weight loss over 12 months was 13 pounds when using a low-carb diet.[19] In a six-month period of time, the average weight loss on this regimen lies between six and 12 pounds for most individuals.[20] And, people have an easy time sticking to a low carb diet. Roughly 80 percent of all people trying to adopt a low carb diet have been able to do so six months or longer.[21]

By all accounts, the low carb diet is safe, effective, and easy to use if weight loss is your primary goal. And at the same time, the low-carb diet also has numerous health benefits.

Specifically, low carb diets help stabilize blood glucose and reduce insulin resistance. Low carb diets are also beneficial in promoting better metabolism and reducing obesity risks.[22] Finally, low-carb diets tend to be easier to adopt because they have less hunger cravings and adequate protein intake as part of their regimen.[23] For all of these reasons, the low-carb diet meets all the criteria for a Diet Stacking approved diet and much more.

The Paleo Diet

This "caveman" approach to healthy dieting is recognized as an effective weight loss diet by many experts. In fact, consuming a diet similar to our paleolithic ancestors has been defined as one of the most rapid weight loss diets around. In surveying a handful of research studies, the average weight loss for individuals on a paleo diet over three months is 11 pounds with a reduction in the waistline in excess of two inches.[24] In addition, because the paleo diet enjoys a high amount of protein, it has also been linked to higher satiety and reduced hunger.[25] Even studies lasting only three weeks involving the paleo diet show weight loss of five pounds on average.[26]

Like many of the diets selected for Diet Stacking, the paleo diet also has other health benefits above and beyond weight loss. In addition to its effects on reducing obesity and fat mass, the paleo diet has also been associated with improved sensitivity to insulin and better blood glucose control.[27] Other studies have also linked the paleo diet to better lipid levels, which reduces cardiovascular risks.[28]

Because of these weight loss and health benefits, and because the paleo diet is simple to adopt, it is an ideal candidate for Diet Stacking.

The Raw Diet

This diet promotes eating organic, fresh, uncooked foods, which are naturally loaded with nutrients and are very healthy. In terms of its ability to help you lose weight, the raw diet has some impressive stats. In reviewing the research, some studies suggest that individuals on the raw diet for three months reduced their body weight by nine percent on average. Another study showed an average weight loss of eight pounds when using the raw diet for seven months. And long-term studies lasting four years have supported that individuals on a raw food diet most commonly have a normal weight for their age and height.[29]

The raw food diet is easy to adopt mainly because of its simple list of foods that can be selected. In addition, it is loaded with nutrients and offers many additional health benefits. In addition to weight loss, the raw diet has been shown to help people with high blood pressure and elevated cholesterol. And it has been associated with better glucose control. These effects have been noted to occur in as little as four weeks while on a raw food diet.[30] As you can see, the raw diet has many advantages while also helping you lose weight fast.

The Elimination Diet

In today's world, a variety of toxins, additives, preservatives, artificial sweeteners, and modified foods exist. At the same time, autoimmune disorders and inflammatory conditions are on the rise. The increased appreciation of how gluten can negatively affect thousands of people supports the need to identify potentially harmful substances in our diet in an effort to achieve better health. By eliminating foods from one's diet that are harmful, a variety of conditions can be resolved ranging from bowel disorders to attention deficit.[31]

While these health benefits are noteworthy, elimination diets are also effective for weight loss. Think about it. When we eat foods that we cannot tolerate, an inflammatory reaction soon follows. This inflammation in the body is associated with a reduced ability of our cells to function well, which affects metabolism, energy levels, and our weight. But nutritionists have noted that by eliminating these substances, we not only feel immediately better, but we can also shed the extra pounds associated with these harmful foods and their side effects.[32] Because of its ability to quickly get to the root of the problem, and provide you with a healthy way to achieve weight loss, the elimination diet has been chosen as an important option for Diet Stacking.

The Anti-Inflammatory Diet

Increasingly, research has shown that chronic inflammation in the body is associated with a number of chronic diseases. For example, research involving nearly 70,000 people who were followed over 16 years has linked chronic inflammation to higher risks for cancer, heart disease and even death.[33] And other research has noted that obesity and diabetes specifically are manifestations of an inflammatory state of the body. In addition to obesity triggering higher levels of inflammation, chronic inflammation also increases weight gain.[34] Understanding this, it is intuitive that the anti-inflammatory diet offers great potential for both weight loss and for overall wellness.

The anti-inflammatory diet takes a perspective that you can lose weight most effectively when your diet provides your body with the proper nutrients while avoiding toxins. Nutrients, including antioxidants, fight chronic inflammation and promote greater weight loss. Toxins that are to be avoided are those substances known to trigger inflammatory and immune reactions in the body leading to weight gain, obesity, and other poor health conditions. As such, the anti-inflammatory diet takes a long-term approach to weight loss and health. Because of these perspectives and values, it has been included as part of the Diet Stacking approved diets.

The Vegan Diet

This popular diet is well known for promoting a diet high in fiber, vegetables and fruit. But in addition to promoting overall wellness, the vegan diet can also help you achieve healthy weight loss when planned appropriately. Research studies have found that those on a vegan diet tend to lose more weight than those on a vegetarian diet.[35] And vegan diets can result in weight loss quite rapidly. One study reported an average of four pounds lost within a month among participants on a vegan diet.[36] Another reports an average of six pounds lost.[37]

Overall, individuals on vegan diets tend to be thinner than the average population, and at the same time, they enjoy an array of great health advantages. For example, vegan diets are associated with lower cholesterol levels, lower blood pressure and reduced risks for cardiovascular disease.[38] Notably, the quality of most vegan diets is superior to others, and the percentage of people who stay on a vegan diet is at least as high as other diets.[39] From a Diet Stacking perspective, vegan diets offer a great way to easily lose weight fast while embracing a healthier way of eating.

The Mediterranean Diet

Among all the Diet Stacking diets, the Mediterranean diet is universally recognized as being one of the healthiest diets available. In addition to being good for your heart and general wellness, the Mediterranean diet offers an excellent approach to regain your ideal weight. Several research studies have demonstrated that individuals on the Mediterranean diet not only lose weight but keep it off. One study showed an average of nine pounds lost that persisted while another showed 6.4 pounds lost from baseline even at two years.[40]

The ability of the Mediterranean diet to promote weight loss is related to its healthy approach to eating and its ability to be easily adopted. Compared to other diets, the Mediterranean diet has a low drop-out rate.[41] And, it is linked to lower blood pressure, lower cholesterol, and reduced risks for heart disease and stroke as well as obesity and diabetes prevention.[42] Among all the diets in the Diet Stack menu of choices, the Mediterranean diet is certainly a "rock star."

The Low-Calorie Diet

This diet offers rapid weight loss through significant calorie restriction. The foundation of this dietary approach stems from groundbreaking research performed in the United Kingdom. Researchers studied obese patients with diabetes and placed them on a low-calorie diet (roughly 700 calories a day) for eight weeks. Within four weeks, the participants lost an average of 10 pounds. And within eight weeks, the average weight loss was 14 pounds. Better yet, even after relaxing the calorie restrictions some, the group was able to keep the weight off.[43]

Given this information, it is evident why the low-calorie diet has been included as an option for Diet Stacking. But you should also appreciate the positive effects this diet can have for those with diabetes and obesity. In fact, a third of the participants in the study effectively reversed their diabetes and were able to stop all medications.[44] This naturally may not apply to all individuals, but the low-calorie diet clearly has health benefits in addition to its impressive weight loss effects.

Different Diet Stacks with Shared Best Practices

As you can see from these brief descriptions of the Diet Stacking approved diets, each offers its own unique approach to weight loss and wellness. However, Diet Stacking embraces some shared approaches that should be applied across all the approved diets. One of the most important of these best practices involves selecting fresh, natural, organic foods whenever possible. At the same time, avoiding refined, processed, and preserved foods is highly recommended as well. Regardless of the Diet Stack approved diet being used, abiding by these rules will boost your health and energy and help you achieve your weight loss goals.

The other recommendation related to the selection of your specific diet stack involves how you combine each of the approved diets. As will be discussed later in the book, common strategies used in combining specific diets will be highlighted. This information is to help guide you in arranging your Diet Stack in a way that will help you achieve your objectives. But at the same time, these are simply recommendations. As you learn more about each of the Diet Stacking approved diets, you will be better able to decide if these recommendations make sense for your unique situation. With this in mind, the following section will describe each Diet Stacking approved diet in greater detail.

SECTION II:
THE DIETS

CHAPTER 4:

THE INTERMITTENT FASTING DIET

For many people, hearing the term fasting might make them cringe. Especially for those of us who love food, fasting sounds horrible! But fasting is not starvation, and modern approaches to fasting (called intermittent fasting) offer a much more appealing (and effective) way to lose weight. Also, researchers are finding that intermittent fasting has many other health benefits in addition to weight loss. From heart health to brain wellness, making an intermittent fasting diet part of your Diet Stack can be an excellent choice.

History of the Intermittent Fasting Diet

Before discussing the history of intermittent fasting diets, one important distinction should be made. Fasting is not starvation. What's the difference? Starvation is involuntary while fasting is not. Intermittent fasting diets allow you to control when you eat and how much food you are permitted during a fast. With this in mind, human starvation dates back to the beginning of humankind while fasting appeared later. But even so, ancient philosophers and healers saw the health benefits of fasting.

Fasting as a practice has been a part of every major religion in the world. For example, Christianity, Buddhism, and Islam all adopt fasting practices as a means to enhance spirituality. At the same time, the ancient Greeks saw fasting as the "physician within." Because the desire to avoid eating when ill was a natural occurrence, Greeks like Hippocrates, Plato, and Aristotle all saw fasting as a healing activity. And even one of our founding fathers, Benjamin Franklin, claimed that rest and fasting were the best medicines in life.[45] If you're thinking about trying an intermittent fasting diet to lose some weight, you're in good company.

More recently, specific intermittent fasting diets (like the 5:2 diet) have become popular. In 2012, journalist and physician Dr. Michael Mosley appeared on the BBC television show *Horizon* advocating the many health benefits of intermittent fasting. Since that time, the so-called "Fast Beach" diet has been embraced by thousands. Not only have these individuals trimmed their waistline, but they've also enjoyed a number of other health advantages in the process. Despite skepticism at first, scientific research is now finding these benefits to be legitimate.[46] This is one reason many experts believe an intermittent fasting diet is among the best diets for weight loss today.

What Is an Intermittent Fasting Diet?

When it comes to weight loss, intermittent fasting can involve a few different options. While religious fasting often requires stopping all food for a period of time, and sometimes even fluids, intermittent fasting diets for weight loss are not usually as extreme. Not only are the periods of fasting time typically shorter, but some food consumption is allowed. What's interesting is that even this level of fasting is associated with tremendous health benefits including weight loss!

For those seeking weight loss, three types of common intermittent fasting diets exist. These include the alternate day fasting, the 5:2 diet, and the time-restricted fasting approach. The alternate day fast is exactly what it sounds like…eat one day, fast the next. The 5:2 diet allows for a normal diet for 5 days each week with 2 days of fasting where calories are reduced to 25 percent of your normal daily intake or less. Lastly, time-restricted fasts require 10 to 16 hours of fasting each day with normal eating otherwise.

Given that your period of time for each diet selected in your Diet Stack is only 3 days, naturally, a 5:2 fasting diet would not be possible. However, a modified version of this using a 2:1 fasting plan with 2 days of fasting and 1 day of normal eating would be reasonable and is what is suggested for your stack.

For the purposes of your Diet Stack, your intermittent fasting will include an intermittent fast on days one and three and regular consumption on day two. During your fasting days, you will consume 500-800 calories depending on your activity level. If you exercise or are moderately active for more than 30 minutes a day, opt for 800 calories. If you don't exercise or are moderately sedentary you should opt for no more than 500 calories on your fasting days. People often freak out a little when you start talking about so few calories. But remember, we're fasting and although we are not giving up all food, we are trying to keep our consumption to a minimum during this time so that we can reap the benefits that fasting provides.

Why Intermittent Fasting Diets Work

When it comes to weight loss, intermittent fasting diets offer some significant advantages. Simply restricting your food intake periodically will reduce the total amount of calories you eat. This will naturally encourage weight loss. But in addition to these effects, intermittent fasting boosts your cells' ability to use glucose and burn energy. By limiting access of food to your body's cells, they become more sensitive to hormones like insulin. Not only does this reduce your risk for developing diabetes, but it also enhances your cells' uptake and use of glucose when available.

In research comparing different weight loss diets, intermittent fasting has been shown to be very effective. Intermittent fasting also offers many other health benefits besides weight loss. Did you know that intermittent fasting helps protect you from developing Alzheimer's disease and Parkinson's disease? Intermittent fasting also enhances your memory and attention. These diets also tend to lower your blood pressure, reduce unhealthy cholesterol levels, and provide some protection against cancers. In addition to helping you lose weight, intermittent fasting reduces inflammation and oxidative stress in the body. All of these effects will help you live a healthier and longer life.

The exact mechanisms by which intermittent fasting helps you rapidly lose weight and become healthier are still being studied. However, it appears that intermittent fasting encourages the cells in your body to be more resilient. This "challenge-recovery" cycle may best align with human history since the steady access to food today is a relatively recent thing. It may just be that our cells are more accustomed to periods of time where glucose levels are lower than other times. If so, then intermittent fasting better mimics situations where human cells may actually thrive.

The Intermittent Fasting Diet as Part of Your Stack

In choosing to include an intermittent fasting diet in your Diet Stack, you will need to decide how to incorporate your 500-800 calories on days 1 and 3. I've found that waiting as long as possible to eat during my fasting days makes the diet much easier. For example on days 1 and 3, I skip breakfast and only consume black coffee, water, tea or sparkling water until lunch and I try to have lunch some time after noon. I will share a typical fasting day with you shortly but first; let's look at some important rules to follow to make the most of your intermittent fast.

- On your non-fasting day, make sure to choose healthy foods and an abundance of vegetables as they will fill you up and help keep you satisfied.
- Don't overcompensate after fasting by binge-eating— this will undermine your chance for success.

- If you are diabetic or pregnant, or if you have an eating disorder, do not do an intermittent fasting program or talk with your doctor before choosing to do so.
- For your fasting days, carbohydrates should be significantly reduced, as they are typically high in calories.
- As always, be sure to drink plenty of water and stay well-hydrated.

In choosing the types of foods you will eat when you are not fasting, an important goal is to select foods that are naturally healthy. This will help you in your weight loss goals, discourage you from binging, and help you achieve better overall health. On your fasting days, your goal should be to reduce your calorie intake to 500 – 800 calories a day. In choosing your "fasting" foods, lean protein, leafy greens and other fibrous vegetables are encouraged. Consume healthy fats in moderation and limit carbohydrates. The following table provides a guide and sample day that can help you in creating an intermittent fasting diet plan that is best for you.

Intermittent Fasting Foods Encouraged When Not Fasting	Intermittent Fasting Foods Encouraged When Partially Fasting
Lean meats and fish are encouraged most of the time	Fish and lean meats are excellent sources of protein and low in calories
Fresh fruits and vegetables of any kind are permissible and encouraged	High fiber vegetables like broccoli, celery, Brussel sprouts, and cauliflower

Intermittent Fasting Foods Encouraged When Not Fasting	Intermittent Fasting Foods Encouraged When Partially Fasting
Low-fat dairy products and eggs	Eggs are also a good source of protein
Healthy fats and oils such as olive oil, nuts, and fats with omega-3s	Avocados, almonds and other nuts that provide healthy fats for calories (in moderation)
Healthy carbohydrates are encouraged with whole grains instead of processed grains	Limit carbohydrates to whole grains and those with high fiber (in moderation)
Beans, legumes, seeds and nuts are all acceptable during non-fasting days	Beans and legumes can be eaten in moderation if low calorie like black beans, peas, and lentils
Smoothies, yogurts and berries are great choices and can provide probiotics	Berries such as blueberries and raspberries can be eaten in moderation

Sample Intermittent Fasting Day

Breakfast: Skip breakfast (black coffee, water, tea or sparkling water until noon)

Lunch: Garden salad with grilled chicken and low calorie non-dairy dressing

Dinner: Chicken and vegetable soup

(Note: Full meal plans are provided in chapters 15, 16 and 17 and recipes are included in Appendix I)

Intermittent Fasting - The Company You Keep

With all the weight loss and health benefits that intermittent fasting provides, it's not surprising that many celebrities endorse it. Of course, these "pop" personalities put their own spin on things. For Hugh Jackman, he routinely sticks to a 16-hour fast each and every day. In addition to helping keep him lean and mean, he admits his diet helps him sleep better as well. Nicole Kidman also chooses a 16-hour fast each day choosing to eat all her meals between 10am and 6pm. And Miranda Kerr has used the 5:2 intermittent fasting diet when she needs to lose weight quickly.[47] These are just a few of the celebrities who have discovered the advantages that intermittent fasting provides.

Intermittent fasting is a great way to boost your weight loss efforts while providing many other long-term health benefits. It's obvious why intermittent fasting diets have so much appeal.

CHAPTER 5:
THE KETOGENIC DIET

In a previous chapter, we talked briefly about the low-carb diet. By comparison, the ketogenic diet is like a low-carb diet to the extreme! In the ketogenic diet, carbohydrates are dropped to a minimum while fats make up most of your body's energy source. Naturally, ketogenic diets help you lose weight, but they work a little differently than low-carb diets. But before you decide if the ketogenic diet is right for you, the following offers some important insights about this popular diet that has been around for more than a century.

History of the Ketogenic Diet

While fasting was a part of ancient Greece, and naturally resulted in dramatic reductions in carbohydrates, the actual ketogenic diet did not really appear until the earliest part of the 20th century. And in fact, the ketogenic diet did not really start out as a weight loss diet at all! Instead, the original ketogenic diet was developed in an effort to sustain better treatment of epilepsy or seizure disorders in the long term.[48] Its weight loss effects were noted much later.

The original physician to label the diet a "ketogenic diet" was Dr. Russell Morse Wilder of the Mayo Clinic around 1923. Previously, fasting diets had been shown to help children with hard-to-control epilepsy, but fasting indefinitely was not an option. Dr. Wilder hoped to prolong these beneficial effects on seizures by using a low carbohydrate, high fat diet. Why? Because this approach had the potential to build up ketones in the body like fasting did. And ketones were the reasons children with epilepsy seemed to improve on these diets.[49]

Overall, the ketogenic diet allows half of all children with seizures to achieve 50 percent improvement in their seizures while a third have 90 percent improvement. But with the introduction of seizure medications, the ketogenic diet fell out of favor after the 1930s. It was not until more recently that the ketogenic diet has had a resurgence. In 1994, the ketogenic diet was again reintroduced as a component of treating children with seizures. And over the last 15 years, its weight loss effects have been readily recognized.[50] As a result, the ketogenic diet is commonly used by thousands today to rapidly lose weight.

What Is a Ketogenic Diet?

A ketogenic diet is essentially a diet that significantly restricts the amount of carbohydrates you eat each day. Instead of getting most of your calories from carbohydrates, which is typical for most people, the ketogenic diet requires most of your body's energy needs to be met by eating fats (and moderate protein). The reduction in carbohydrates is what triggers your body to start metabolizing fats in your body, and this is what can trigger significant weight loss.

The classic ketogenic diet adopts a ratio of 4-to-1, which means you receive four times the amount of your body's energy needs from fats when compared to both proteins and carbohydrates. For most people, that means the amount of carbohydrates you can have on a ketogenic diet is less than 20 grams a day.[51] While some modified ketogenic diets allow 20 to 50 grams of carbohydrates daily, the abbreviated use of the ketogenic diet in a Diet Stack should align better with a 20 to 30 gram per day limit of carbs.

So, what does all of this mean in terms of actual foods? Many people like the ketogenic diet because of the foods you can enjoy on a regular basis. While breads, pastas, and pizza are off the list, fatty meats are encouraged. For example, grass-fed beef, beef brisket, pork shoulder, bacon, and salmon are perfectly acceptable choices on a ketogenic diet. Other ketogenic diet foods include leafy vegetables, high-fiber vegetables, avocado, and nuts, seeds and healthy oils. For some people looking to lose weight, the ketogenic diet sounds pretty appealing.

Why Ketogenic Diets Work

The reason why ketogenic diets are attractive is that they can help get rid of the stored fat we have in our bodies. By drastically reducing the amounts of carbs we eat, our body must begin either breaking down fats in our bodies or using dietary fats for energy. This process is called ketosis, which simply means fats are metabolized into ketones. Instead of your body metabolizing sugars and carbs for energy, your body adapts to breaking down fats as an alternative.

Ketones that result from a ketogenic diet include molecules like acetone, acetoacetate, and beta-hydroxybutyrate. These molecules are not only used for energy but they also are believed to be the reason ketogenic diets help children with seizures.[52] In terms of weight loss, ketogenic diets help you shed the pounds simply by shifting how your body's cells go about meeting their energy needs. Once the ketogenic "shift" occurs, losing weight from stored fat in the body becomes more efficient and easier.

According to some experts, this ketogenic shift can occur as early as two days after beginning a ketogenic diet, however, this can vary from person to person. In addition to promoting rapid weight loss, the ketogenic diet has other potential benefits. This includes better glucose control, improved mood, better energy, and more focused mental clarity. While nausea, fatigue, constipation and bad breath may occur early after beginning the diet, these usually dissipate quickly.[53] As long as you can live without your carbs, the ketogenic diet has many advantages for those of us pursuing weight loss.

The Ketogenic Diet as Part of Your Stack

Following a ketogenic diet as part of your Diet Stack is fairly straightforward, but there are a few rules and guidelines that are notably important. Indeed, the ketogenic diet offers a wide variety of foods to be eaten, but the diet does require that you restrict your carbohydrates significantly. Failure to do so will defeat the purpose (and benefits) of a ketogenic diet. If you choose the ketogenic diet as one of your Diet Stacking approved diets, you will only need to maintain this restriction for the 3-day period. The following offers some best practices during this time when it comes to ketogenic dieting.

- Carbohydrates should total only 20 to 30 grams per day
- Watch out for high-carb vegetables and fruits like potatoes, carrots, oranges, and bananas
- A fat-to-protein/carb ratio should be about 4-to-1 in terms of calories
- Continue to eat a reasonable number of calories based on your height, gender, and level of activity
- Drink ample amounts of water in order to reduce unwanted side effects from ketones

In addition to understanding the basic guidelines of a ketogenic diet, it also helps to know major categories of foods that are allowed and ones that should be avoided. Plenty of food options exist with a ketogenic diet, but knowing which foods to avoid is very important given how common they are in our diets.

Ketogenic Diet Foods Allowed	Ketogenic Diet Foods to Avoid
All types of meats with fatty cuts preferred	All grains and bread products
Fatty seafood selections like salmon, catfish, trout, etc.	Most fruits including citrus, bananas, plums, mango, pears, apples and grapes
High fat dairy products such as creams	Skim milk products and low-fat dairy
Cheeses and eggs	Sugars and most sweeteners like honey
Most fats and oils including butter, ghee, coconut oil, lard, mayonnaise	Some oils such as peanut, canola, sunflower, and sesame seed oil
Leafy and high fiber vegetables including cabbage, spinach, lettuce, broccoli, cauliflower, asparagus and zucchini	Root vegetables such as carrots, potatoes, beets, turnips and yams
All types of nuts including nut milks	All beans and legumes
Rare and limited use of select berries such as blackberries, blueberries and raspberries	Alcohol with particular attention to higher carb drinks like beer and sweet wines

When following the ketogenic diet, you should also continue to track your calories each day. Fats provide a total of nine calories per gram while carbs and proteins only provide four calories per gram. This means that the higher fat content of a ketogenic diet will allow you to meet your body's energy needs with fewer grams of food since the fat ratio is higher. To truly benefit from a ketogenic diet, keep track of your daily calories to make sure you do not "overshoot" your body's needs. This will give you the best chance for effective weight loss success!

Sample Ketogenic Day

<u>Day 1</u>

Breakfast: Baked egg and avocado

Lunch: Lettuce wrapped BLT

Snack: 10-15 Almonds

Dinner: Almond-crusted chicken with steamed asparagus

> *(Note: Full meal plans are provided in chapters 15, 16 and 17 and recipes are included in Appendix I)*

Ketogenic Dieting - The Company You Keep

It's highly likely that you know plenty of people who have realized tremendous success with a ketogenic diet. Therefore, you probably aren't surprised that several celebrities in the spotlight strongly support the ketogenic diet for weight loss and health. For example, Vanessa Hudgens not only likes adding bacon to her morning breakfast as part of a ketogenic diet, but she acknowledges that the ketogenic diet gives her steady energy throughout her day. Even sports celebrities like Tim Tebow and LeBron James have embraced the ketogenic diet to shed some pounds while achieving optimal athletic performance.

In selecting the ketogenic diet as part of your Diet Stack, you may want to be strategic in choosing other Diet Stacking approved diets in your stack. Because the weight loss benefits of the ketogenic diet rely on the ketogenic "shift" in your body's metabolism, it can be paired well with low carb diets, paleo diets, and intermittent fasting diets. Take this into consideration when evaluating which Diet Stacking approved diets you might want to include in your stack. If the ketogenic diet is one that sounds appealing, you are not alone. The ketogenic diet has helped many people lose weight, and it can work for you too!

CHAPTER 6:
THE LOW-CARB DIET

Low-carbohydrate diets have been around a long time, and most of us at one time or another have "cut the carbs" in an effort to lose weight. But opinions about low-carb diets have fluctuated over the years. At times, experts have encouraged low-carb diets only to be followed later by them falling out of favor. Like most weight loss diets, the truth lies somewhere in between, but without question, the low-carb diet can be a very effective diet for sustained weight loss and health. Exploring the low-carb diet in greater detail can shed some light on why this diet can be a smart choice for your Diet Stack program.

History of the Low-Carb Diet

Low-carb diets are nothing new. In fact, some medical reports show the use of a low-carb diet to treat diabetes dating back to the 1700s.[54] However, the low-carb diet really gained popularity in the mid-19th century when William Banting, whose claim to fame was being the coffin-maker for the Duke of Wellington, discovered the weight loss benefits of eating fewer carbs. By cutting out bread, butter, beer, sugar and potatoes from his diet, Banting lost over 50 pounds within a year's time! Having suffered obesity throughout his life, and after numerous attempts to lose weight through other diet and lifestyle changes, he finally found the answer by lowering his carbohydrate intake.[55]

Let's now fast forward to the latter part of the 20th century. In 1972, Dr. Robert C. Atkins released his book, *Dr. Atkin's Diet Revolution*. Amidst a craze of low-fat diets being promoted by government and nutritional organizations alike to reduce heart disease, Dr. Atkin's suggested that a low-carb approach was better.[56] Since then, numerous scientific studies have shown that higher carbohydrate diets lead to a number of health problems. In addition to weight issues, higher carb diets promote obesity and diabetes, both of which are current epidemics in our world. While the low-carb diet gained traction in the 1980s and 1990s, it continues to be well supported by science today.[57]

What Is a Low-Carb Diet?

Carbohydrates, or carbs, are often referred to as starches or sugars. At the same time, whole grains and fiber are actually carbs as well. The difference among these carbs involves how quickly they are absorbed into our bodies. For example, sugars and refined carbs are easily absorbed and cause rapid increases in blood sugar levels. These are often found in processed and sweetened foods, fruits, and juices. In contrast, complex carbs and fibers take longer to be metabolized and are healthier. These more complex carbs are found in whole grains and in some vegetables.

So, what makes a diet "low" in carbs? In order to answer this, you first need to know what is considered a normal amount of dietary carbs for the average person. Most non-weight loss diets that promote health and wellness suggest that carbs should comprise 45 to 65 percent of your total calories. For the average adult, this usually means about 200 grams of carbohydrates each day. Therefore, anything less than this could be considered a low-carb diet. But things aren't quite that simple.

Low-carb diets are broken down into different categories. For example, diets receiving 26 to 45 percent of their calories from carbs are called "moderately low" carb diets while those less than 26 percent are considered "very low-carb" diets. But any diet that is comprised of 100 grams or less of daily carbohydrate intake can be considered low-carb. Diets with fewer than 20 percent of your calories coming from carbs are often termed as ketogenic diets. For stacking purposes, the low-carb diet should follow guidelines of no more than 100 grams of daily carbohydrate intake.

Why Low-Carb Diets Work

Because carbs are converted to blood sugars rather quickly, eating carbohydrates can naturally trigger a rise in your blood glucose level after a meal. This, in turn, triggers the release of insulin. And insulin promotes cells in your body to absorb the glucose for energy. However, when excess glucose is floating around, insulin also promotes converting glucose into fat for energy storage. Therefore, low-carb diets naturally reduce the chance that glucose will be turned into fat.

But you want to lose weight, not simply avoid additional weight gain. Don't worry…low-carb diets help here too. First of all, low-carb diets have been shown to reduce hunger and improve satiety. With fewer carbs around, blood sugar levels are less likely to fluctuate. A more stable blood sugar level means fewer cravings and episodes of hunger. In addition, by replacing carbs with protein, your body can produce its own glucose from stored fat easier. This helps not only reduce your hunger, but it also helps get rid of that excess weight.[58]

Low-carb diets offer many health benefits in addition to helping you lose weight. Lowering your carbs helps stabilize blood sugar levels and improve cholesterol profiles at the same time. In addition, low-carb diets have been shown to be particularly effective if you are significantly overweight.[59] There's a reason low-carb diets have been around for centuries, so including a low-carb diet as part of your diet stack is well supported by both research and experience.

The Low-Carb Diet as Part of Your Stack

Choosing a low-carb diet as part of your Diet Stack is a great choice! But in order to do this effectively, you need to know which foods can be included in your low-carb meal plan and which ones should be avoided. In addition, as part of your stack your three-day low-carb diet should follow specific guidelines as follows:

- Keep total daily carbs less than 100 grams a day (or less than 25 percent of total calories)

- Avoid simple sugars and refined carbohydrates (includes fruits and fruit juices)
- Choose high fiber and complex carbohydrates for dietary carbs selected
- Replace calories lost from carbohydrates preferentially with proteins rather than fats

As a general rule, lean meats, vegetables that grow above ground, and unsweetened dairy can all be included in your low-carb diet meal plan. In contrast, breads, pastas, rice, beans, potatoes, and most fruits need to be limited. Even if you don't have time to plan a specific meal, these basic rules offer some general guidelines for a low-carb diet.

Low-Carb Diet Foods Allowed	Low-Carb Diet Foods to Avoid
Lean meats and fish	Breads and cereals
Leafy green vegetables	Pastas
Cauliflower and broccoli	Rice and refined grains
Nuts and seeds	Beans
Olive oil, avocado oil, coconut oil	Potatoes and starchy root vegetables
Unsweetened dairy products such as milk and yogurt	Fruit juices, sodas and sugar-sweetened beverages
Cheeses	Processed foods/products with added sugar
Select fruits (in moderation) – apples, strawberries, pears, and blueberries	Most fruits – bananas, oranges, pineapple, peaches, plums

While these general guidelines are helpful, knowing which foods contain carbs and the number of carb grams per serving allows you to better stick to your low-carb diet. A number of carb calculators are available on the Internet, including one offered by WebMD (https://www.webmd.com/diet/healthtool-food-calorie-counter). Likewise, "carb counter" apps are also available to assist in your low-carb meal planning. These are easy-to-use tools that make it simple to plan your low-carb diet stacking meals.

Sample Low-Carb Day

Day 1

Breakfast: Veggie omelet and two strips bacon

Lunch: Greek salad with grilled salmon

Snack: 1oz string cheese

Dinner: Rosemary chicken with steamed broccoli

(Note: Full meal plans are provided in chapters 15, 16 and 17 and recipes are included in Appendix I)

Low-Carb Dieting – The Company You Keep

When it comes to low-carb dieting, dozens of celebrities and high-profile personalities support its effectiveness for both health and weight loss. For example, actress Courteney Cox avoids carbs and chooses to eat primarily lean meats and vegetables to keep her stellar physique. Similarly, Alyssa Milano discovered the weight loss benefits of low-carb dieting after having her second child. And Halle Berry is a vocal advocate of low-carb diets, especially for those with diabetes like herself.

Low-carb diets are not only effective in promoting steady weight loss, but they are also very effective in reducing your risk for a number of unwanted health conditions. And after being on a low-carb diet, you may well find those pesky cravings and hunger attacks disappear. Including a low-carb diet in your Diet Stack is a great way to lose weight and rest assured that you are eating healthy at the same time.

CHAPTER 7:

THE PALEO DIET

The Paleolithic period extended from 2.6 million years ago until about 10,000 years ago. Our species, as it is known today, has been around about 20,000 years. Thus, some of our human ancestors lived during paleolithic times when the only means for securing food was through hunting and gathering. No fast-food restaurants, no processed foods, no agricultural farms—just simple, natural foods that existed in nature.

Today, many choose to eat a Paleo diet, which attempts to mimic the "caveman" diet of our earlier ancestors. With the assumption that modern diets contribute to chronic diseases like heart disease, diabetes, and obesity, the Paleo diet offers an alternative in the pursuit of better health. But at the same time, the Paleo diet has also been used as an effective weight loss diet. For these reasons, the Paleo diet is included as an option for your Diet Stack selections.

History of the Paleo Diet

Unlike many of the other Diet Stacking choices, the Paleo diet is a relatively recent approach to weight loss and health. The concept of the Paleo diet was originally developed in the 1990s by Dr. Loren Cordain. As the founder of the Paleo diet and the one who coined the term, Dr. Cordain acknowledged how rapidly the human diet has changed in comparison to the evolution of mankind. At the same time, he appreciated the rapid rise in a number of chronic illnesses throughout the world. These observations led him to consider an alternative to the highly-processed, agriculturally-driven diet most of us eat today.[60]

Notably, the foods accessible to most of us today come from large agricultural operations that generate various crops and foods. These foodstuffs are often processed for easy shipping, storage, handling and purchase. Also, the addition of preservatives and other chemicals are common today throughout the process as well. Despite food production being routine today, it's actually relatively new. In fact, the industrial and agricultural revolutions are not even 200 years old!

Dr. Cordain noted that while these "advances" in foods have occurred in a relatively fast manner, the human DNA has changed only about 0.2 percent over tens of thousands of years.[61] It therefore seems quite logical that our digestive, immune, and other body systems are poorly equipped to handle today's foods. By adopting a more primitive, natural, and basic approach to eating, we have a chance to reclaim better health and rid ourselves of many of the chronic illnesses common in today's societies.

What Is a Paleo Diet?

When thinking about a Paleo diet, think about what would have been available to our prehistoric cousins. Of course, many of these foods are not likely to be on the shelf at your grocery store, but trying to choose foods closest to what was available in those times is what's important. The Paleo diet is based on the hunter-gatherer perspective. Foods that could be naturally hunted or gathered in the wild are those that our digestive systems can best tolerate.

So, what are some examples of foods that may not be well tolerated in our diets today? An obvious example is gluten. Grains are not part of a Paleo diet because these foods require processing of naturally occurring wheat. No one ate such foodstuffs in Paleolithic times because agricultural and food processing didn't exist. So, gluten wasn't a natural part of the human diet during prehistoric times. Other examples of foods absent include most dairy products, sugary treats, and processed meats.

A Paleo diet, therefore, includes foods that hunters and gatherers may come across during their search for food in the wild. Grass-fed meats, fish, and seafood are naturally occurring. Likewise, fruits, vegetables, and nuts are also readily available in nature and may be eaten as part of a Paleo diet plan. By choosing these types of foods, not only can you enjoy better digestion but healthier weight as well.

Why Paleo Diets Work

The rationale behind the Paleo diet involves trying to align our diets with our bodies' needs. The foods included in a Paleo diet are not only unprocessed, whole foods, but they are also highly nutritious. Paleo diets offer natural foods that provide an array of vitamins, minerals and antioxidants.

Many of these nutritious substances may be lost in processing, and therefore, poor health may result.

Paleo diets offer foods that can also be more easily digested. Naturally occurring fruits, vegetables, seafood, and grass-fed meats have been part of the human diet for thousands of centuries. Digestive problems are therefore less likely to occur because our bodies are used to these foods. The prevalence of conditions like diabetes, obesity, gluten sensitivity, and food allergies are all affected by diet and digestive changes. By adopting a Paleo diet, you give your body a chance to digest meals more effectively.

Lastly, Paleo diets also help you lose weight. Without the added sugars, processed carbohydrates, and high-fat dairy products, achieving a healthy weight is a natural side effect of a Paleo diet. While watching your overall calories is still recommended for the purpose of losing weight, a Paleo diet promotes healthy weight. In fact, many people choose a Paleo diet for this reason alone.

The Paleo Diet as Part of Your Stack

Overall, the Paleo Diet is relatively straightforward. Think like a prehistoric cave-dweller, and you should be fine! Like any healthy, nutritious diet, a variety of foods should be included since variety offers the best way to get all the vitamins, minerals and nutrients your body requires. But in addition, the following guidelines for a Paleo diet can be followed to help you during your three-day Paleo Diet.

- General rules for food selections are those foodstuffs that occur naturally and are in the wild
- Fruits, vegetables, nuts, seafood, and grass-fed meats are common foods included
- Peanuts are not considered a nut but instead a legume and should be avoided
- Daily calorie counts are still important for weight loss purposes
- Only natural sweeteners like honey and maple syrup should be included

Unlike some of the other Diet Stacking approved diets, the Paleo diet has more generous options when it comes to the amount of carbohydrates and fats in your meal plan. For this reason, it is important to monitor your overall daily calories. With this in mind, the following offers food options that should be included or avoided as part of your Paleo Diet meal plan.

Paleo Diet Foods Allowed	Paleo Diet Foods to Avoid
Grass-fed meats, fish and shellfish	All processed meats
Most all vegetables	Vegetables with high levels of starch like potatoes
Most all fruits	All types of grains
Eggs	All dairy products, cheese, etc.
All types of nuts (excluding peanuts)	Beans, legumes and peanuts

Paleo Diet Foods Allowed	Paleo Diet Foods to Avoid
Honey, maple syrup and other natural, unprocessed sweeteners	All refined sugars, artificial sweeteners
Naturally occurring seeds	Salted, processed or preserved foods
Healthy oils like olive oil, avocado oil and coconut oil	Alcohol of all types

In considering which diets to combine with a Paleo diet in your Diet Stack, several good options exist and will be discussed in greater detail in section three: Finding Your Stack. In general, the weight-loss aspect of the Paleo diet reflects the amount of overall calorie restriction you choose. Regardless, the Paleo diet has been shown to enhance your health as well as promote weight loss.

Sample Paleo Day

Breakfast: 2 hardboiled eggs and small fruit salad

Lunch: Grilled chicken breast, side salad

Snack: 10-15 Almonds

Dinner: Grass fed steak and steamed asparagus

(Note: Full meal plans are provided in chapters 15, 16 and 17 and recipes are included in Appendix I)

Paleo Dieting – The Company You Keep

Despite Paleo diets being a relative newcomer to the diet scene, they are not without their celebrity endorsers. Several well-known personalities recommend Paleo diets not only for health but for also achieving that "hot" body. For example, Matthew McConaughey sticks to a Paleo diet at least 90 percent of the time. Likewise, Jessica Biel regularly eats a Paleo meal plan because she enjoys the way it makes her feel lean and healthy. And Miley Cyrus, known for being gluten and dairy sensitive, is a strong supporter of a Paleo lifestyle.[62]

In today's age where processed foods are everywhere, getting back to natural foods using a Paleo diet makes a lot of sense. Natural foods are much easier to digest, and they offer less stress to our system. And by including a variety of different natural foods, Paleo diets offer great nutrition and promote healthy weight loss. Including a Paleo diet in your Diet Stack can help you attain a variety of health goals and shed some excess weight.

CHAPTER 8:

THE RAW DIET

Heating and processing various foods has been recognized as being potentially harmful when it comes to optimal health. Unlike fresh, uncooked, whole foods that are packed with vitamins and nutrients, cooked foods may lose some of their nutritional value. As a result, many people believe a raw food diet is one of the healthiest diets. And likewise, a raw diet is great for weight loss. Because of the raw diet's strong health and weight loss benefits, it is also included as a dietary option in your Diet Stack. And for thousands, "raw" has become a way of life.

History of the Raw Diet

The raw diet had its origins around the beginning of the 20th century. Of course, eating raw fruits and vegetables has always been in vogue, sometimes by necessity. Just ask any cave dweller! But the raw diet's modern appeal as a health and weight loss diet has been more recent. In a book published in 1903 entitled *Uncooked Foods and How to Use Them*, Mr. and Mrs. Eugene Christian highlighted how raw foods could cure stomach problems. This book not only provided recipe instructions but identified how raw foods might help your digestion.

In 1938, nutritionist and physician Maximillian Bircher-Benner released his book, *The Prevention of Incurable*

Diseases. He believed raw foods and carbohydrates were much healthier than cooked foods and high levels of protein. In essence, Bircher-Benner believed the lack of whole foods and the destruction of food nutrients from heating was the main cause of most illnesses. In fact, he came to this conclusion after treating his own condition of jaundice with fresh apples and other raw foods.[63]

In recent decades, raw foods have gained additional support from a number of nutrition experts. This group includes Dr. Joel Fuhrman, the well-known physician and nutritionist. As foods have been increasingly processed, manipulated, and prepared through various measures, many associate a rise in illnesses with these dietary changes. Getting back to raw foods is believed to provide better long-term health and longevity. And it has been well recognized as an effective weight loss diet. Thus, the raw diet continues to be quite popular.

What Is a Raw Diet?

A raw diet is exactly what you think it is…raw food. Foods that can be included in a raw diet are those that have not been processed, cooked, microwaved or irradiated in any way. Likewise, foods that are genetically modified, chemically treated, or heated above 115 degrees Fahrenheit are not considered raw either. Given these criteria, the actual foods permitted as part of a raw diet are rather limited. These include primarily fresh fruits, vegetables, nuts, seeds and few raw meats that are safe to eat.

Essentially, a raw diet is a plant-based diet. While some select raw meats such as sashimi might be included, the vast majority of raw diet meals consist of fruits, vegetables and nuts. In fact, 75 to 80 percent of a raw diet ends up being from fresh plants. What's notably absent from a raw diet? Anything pasteurized, processed, or cooked. Therefore, a raw diet will not include any pasteurized dairy products, cooked animal meats, or even pastas and breads. You can appreciate why some people struggle with such a diet over time.

As a weight loss diet, however, a raw diet is excellent. Since many foods in a raw diet are naturally low in calories, most people end up eating about half the calories that they would normally eat. At the same time, many raw foods have high fiber content. This means that you feel less hungry despite eating fewer calories. These benefits, in addition to the higher nutritious value of a raw diet, account for its continued popularity despite its significant food restrictions.

Why Raw Diets Work

So, why do raw diets work? Based on several studies, raw diets appear to offer many health and weight benefits. Some research suggests that people on raw diets live longer while others show raw diets reduce your risk for some types of cancers. Likewise, some research suggests raw diets improve heart health and blood sugar control.[64] Given these scientific findings, it appears that proponents of raw diets may be onto something.

The basic premise of a raw diet is that essential vitamins, minerals, and nutrients are better preserved in foods when they are not exposed to heat or chemical processing. Indeed, heating some foods has been associated with the production of carcinogens or may destroy the structure of vitamins, minerals and proteins in the food.[65] By eating raw foods, you can therefore provide your body with better nutrition, which in turn provides better health.

Certainly, better health is a goal we all want to achieve, and part of good health involves a healthy weight. Some of the health benefits attributed to a raw diet involve its ability to help you lose excess weight. You might say that raw diets provide a one-two punch when it comes to health. On the one hand, a raw diet gives your body exactly what it needs to stay healthy. And secondly, it helps you maintain a healthy weight that reduces the chance of many other illnesses. Making a raw diet a part of your Diet Stack therefore offers you some serious advantages.

The Raw Diet Stack

By choosing a raw diet as part of your Diet Stack, you will certainly save time in cooking and meal preparation! Many of the foods included in a raw diet can be eaten as they are or combined rather quickly, which gives you more time for other activities. It is important to be prepared, however, and some simple pieces of advice can go a long way in helping you adhere to a raw diet and reap its benefits.

- Keep plenty of fresh fruits, nuts, and seeds on hand for quick snacks throughout the day
- A blender and/or food processor can be highly valuable
- Buy fresh produce that is organic and without any chemical or preservatives
- Do not eat raw rhubarb, cassava, taro, or sprouted potatoes, which can contain toxins when raw
- Be safe if you choose to eat raw meats, fish or unpasteurized dairy

The following table provides a list of foods that may be included in your Raw Diet Stack as well as those that need to be avoided. In essence, anything heated, processed or refined should not be included while raw, natural, fresh, organic foods are perfectly fine. However, some caution is important when considering some raw foods like meats and select vegetables. Using this table will help you determine which foods are best to include in your Raw Diet Stack.

Raw Diet Stack Foods Allowed	Raw Diet Stack Foods to Avoid
Organic fresh fruits of all kinds	No foods heated over 115 degrees F
Organic fresh vegetables of all kinds, some select raw meats such as fish/sashimi	Raw cassava, taro, rhubarb and sprouted potatoes
Raw nuts and seeds	Processed foods and beverages
Raw sprouted and soaked grains such as oats, millet, barley, and buckwheat	Pastas, breads, refined grains including flour

Raw Diet Stack Foods Allowed	Raw Diet Stack Foods to Avoid
Olive oil, coconut oil and almond butter	Process oils, butters, fats
Raisins, dates, dried coconut, and other dried fruits	Refined sugar, pastries, and junk foods
Fresh herbs, natural sea salt, and apple cider vinegar for seasoning	Iodized salt, processed seasonings and herbs
Wine is permissible if organic and without preservatives	Beer and spirits as well as caffeine

As described, many people on a raw diet will naturally eat fewer calories simply because most raw foods are less caloric overall. Like any plant-based diet, the ability to reduce your daily calories and feel more satiated is much easier. But at the same time, it is important to keep measuring your daily calorie intake if weight loss is your goal. This will not only help you keep track of your dieting but also ensure you are getting enough calories to stay healthy.

Sample Raw Diet Day

Day 1

Breakfast: Green Juice

Lunch: Kale, walnut and pear salad

Snack: Trail mix and sliced apple

Dinner: Raw zucchini "spaghetti" with avocado pesto

(Note: Full meal plans are provided in chapters 15, 16 and 17 and recipes are included in Appendix I)

Raw Dieting – The Company You Keep

Whether you choose to eat a raw diet as part of your Diet Stack or make it a part of your ongoing lifestyle, you will have plenty of fellow raw diet advocates. Many celebrity superstars recommend a raw diet, and their youthfulness and physiques alone are enough to grab your attention. For example, Madonna chooses a fairly strict raw-food diet most of the time and has for decades. Demi Moore likewise encourages a raw diet stating it makes her not only feel well-nourished but also incredibly healthy. And Woody Harrelson has maintained his physique by only eating raw foods and avoiding all animal products.[66]

For many people who eat a raw diet long term, the benefits for health and weight loss become obvious. Even if the occasional non-raw food is included, the benefits of the raw diet are still impressive. If eating a raw diet sounds too difficult or limited for you, remember each diet in the Diet Stacking program only last for three days—a period of time that most of us could adhere to rather easily.

CHAPTER 9:

THE ELIMINATION DIET

When it comes to dieting, losing excess weight is probably your primary motivator. But for many people, weight loss is not the only concern when it comes to selecting a diet. In fact, over 15 million people suffer from some type of food allergy or intolerance. In addition, many individuals are not even aware their diet is the cause of their complaints. Therefore, depending on your unique situation, you might consider an elimination diet as part of your Diet Stack. As you will learn, an elimination diet can help you in your weight loss efforts while potentially making you feel healthier in other ways.

History of the Elimination Diet

Elimination diets don't have an extensive history like many other diets discussed in this book. In fact, eliminating or avoiding specific foods in an effort to lose weight or to feel better was only conceptualized in the last century. The increase in processed foods, wheat, dairy, corn and soy has been associated with an increase in food allergies. In fact, according to recent reports from the Centers for Disease Control and Prevention, roughly 4 percent of the population now have some kind of food allergy.[67]

One of the first people to suggest eliminating foods in an effort to promote health was a California-based physician back in the 1920s. Dr. Albert Row was dissatisfied with the accuracy of allergy skin testing. So, he recommended that people cut foods from their diet for a period of time to see if they had a food allergy to a specific food or not. He described a condition that he called "allergic epigastric syndrome," that occurred when people developed food allergies. Interestingly, this syndrome had all the same features that we associate with food intolerance today. Through strict oversight of one's diet, Dr. Rowe believed specific foods could be identified that caused various symptoms, and he believed this was much better than other types of allergy testing overall.[68]

Since Dr. Rowe's initial description of an elimination diet, hundreds of healthcare professionals have now embraced this approach to better health. Given the millions who are affected by various food intolerances, it's not surprising that the elimination diet has grown in popularity. But the elimination diet has also been used by many for weight loss as well. In addition to diet restrictions that might help you shed some pounds, the elimination diet can also reduce inflammation in your digestive system and body that could potentially boost your metabolism. For this reason, many people now appreciate Dr. Rowe's insights from decades ago.

What Is an Elimination Diet?

The elimination diet is exactly what it sounds like…you eliminate foods to see if your body responds favorably. But in addition to wanting to lose weight, you should know about some of the more common symptoms associated with food allergies and intolerances. Certainly, indigestion, stomach cramps, and other intestinal problems can indicate an intolerance to food. But several other less obvious symptoms can indicate a food problem as well. For example, achy muscle pains, headaches, poor concentration, and even fatigue can be symptoms related to a food allergy. In fact, difficulty losing weight can even be related to specific food allergies.

An elimination diet essentially cuts those foods most likely to be causing your symptoms out of your diet for a period of time. In doing so, your body has the chance to recover and improve. With this in mind, an elimination diet involves four simple steps…planning, avoiding, challenging, and maintaining. During the planning phase, you collect information about your diet and symptoms using a food diary. By recording what you eat, how much you eat, the timing of your symptoms, and other relevant information, you can better identify which foods you want to cut from your diet first. This provides you the best opportunity to achieve the weight loss and health goals you want.

After the planning phase, the elimination diet then involves avoiding the foods you identified while monitoring your weight and other symptoms. For most people, symptoms should improve over several days. If this occurs, then you slowly add a single food type back, one at a time (called the challenging phase), to see if symptoms come back. You will know if a specific food is causing a problem within three days of starting it back. The elimination diet then proceeds through this trial-and-error approach until you are able to define an overall diet best for you. And in the process, you may very well find you are better able to achieve the ideal weight you want!

For the purpose of your diet stack, however, the elimination diet will take on a slightly simpler approach. Since your elimination diet will last only three days, you will be asked to cut the five foods that often cause the most issues for people: sugar, wheat, dairy, soy, and alcohol.

Why Elimination Diets Work

From the perspective of food allergies and intolerances, it seems pretty clear why an elimination diet works. Simply remove the offending item from your diet, and your symptoms will get better. But identifying a single food allergy is not always so easy, especially when the particular substance may be hidden in a variety of foods. People with gluten allergies are well aware that gluten can be hidden in a number of foods that might not necessarily be recognized as wheat-based. The same goes for lactose, casein, and soy, which are also ingredients in a variety of foods.

Elimination diets work because they take a structured approach to avoiding specific foods most likely to cause your complaints and then reintroducing isolated foods back one at a time. While this explains why most food allergy symptoms respond, it may not be readily apparent how an elimination diet allows weight loss. Though precise mechanisms are not well understood, it is appreciated that food allergies trigger inflammation and immune system reactions throughout the body. As a result, your metabolism may be affected, and your symptoms may affect your appetite, food choices, and activity level. Depending on these reactions, you might experience weight gain as a result. Therefore, an elimination diet can not only help you reduce the amount of food you are eating overall, but it may also improve your health.

The Elimination Diet as Part of Your Stack

With an elimination diet, different levels of intensity may be considered. For example, some people choose a simple elimination diet that only removes one or two foods at a time. More complex elimination diets avoid several foods at once. As mentioned earlier, for the purposes of your stack, you will eliminate sugar, wheat, dairy, soy, and alcohol. The following offers some recommended strategies to help you if you select the elimination diet as part of your Diet Stack.

- Eliminate the selected foods throughout the entire three-day elimination diet
- Read all labels carefully to ensure you are truly avoiding the identified foods
- Be extra careful when eating at restaurants or when dining at friends' homes
- Drink plenty of water to stay well hydrated

Although elimination diets typically last for several weeks as people discover which foods may be negatively affecting them, you can benefit from eliminated foods that typically cause the most damage. Even just three days without sugar, wheat, dairy, soy, and alcohol can make a huge difference in how you feel, how much energy you have and how well you sleep.

The following is a list of foods you should avoid and foods you can include while doing the elimination diet. Typically the foods you choose to avoid are specific to your individual symptoms however, for the purposes of your diet stack the following table details the foods to avoid and foods that are allowed.

Elimination Diet Foods Allowed	Elimination Diet Foods to Avoid
All fruit (in moderation)	Sugar
Nut-based milks like almond milk	Dairy products and foods containing casein and lactose
Legumes of all kinds	Wheat, rye, barley, etc.
Rice, quinoa, and buckwheat	Soy and soy byproducts
All vegetables, fresh and organic preferred	Peanuts (optional)
Almonds, cashews, pecans and various seeds	Alcohol
Fish and lean poultry	Red meat (optional)

A specific note regarding weight-loss goals should also be made when it comes to the elimination diet. Certainly, improving your health by avoiding foods that trigger food allergies has the potential to help you achieve a more ideal weight. But in addition, paying attention to calories consumed on the elimination diet remains important in an effort to achieve weight-loss goals. Therefore, be sure to choose healthy options while avoiding foods you think are causing problems. This will give you the best chance to succeed in achieving your overall goals!

Sample Elimination Diet Day

Breakfast: Overnight oats and blueberries

Lunch: Four-bean salad

Snack: 10-15 Almonds and 1 pear

Dinner: White chicken stew

(Note: Full meal plans are provided in chapters 15, 16 and 17 and recipes are included in Appendix I)

Elimination Dieting – The Company You Keep

Unlike other popular weight-loss diets, celebrities may not tout the elimination diet as the diet that "rocked their world." But plenty of well-known personalities have realized the benefits an elimination diet provides. These benefits not only include health improvements but also weight loss. For example, Khloe Kardashian realized how much healthier she felt after completely eliminating cheese and milk from her diet. Megan Fox also eliminated dairy from her diet. As she describes, if you want to lose weight, get rid of the dairy! And Gisele Bundchen and Tom Brady stick to a diet that aligns perfectly well with the approved foods described in an elimination diet.[69]

The elimination diet may not be the best option for everyone. But if you believe your weight gain or other symptoms could be related to your diet, then the elimination diet is an excellent choice. For example, a raw diet, an intermittent fasting diet, or a low-calorie diet might be great choices to combine with an elimination diet in your Diet Stack. If you feel better after the 3-days on the elimination diet, you may decide to follow a stricter elimination protocol after your stack is completed to find out which of the five foods we eliminated is negatively affecting you. By making these selections wisely, you will be better able to detect a specific food that might be contributing to your weight gain or complaints.

CHAPTER 10:

THE ANTI-INFLAMMATORY DIET

Throughout the world today, a variety of chronic diseases are on the rise. Conditions like obesity, diabetes, heart disease and cancer as well as Alzheimer's disease are becoming increasingly common. What do all of these health conditions have in common? Each is linked to chronic inflammation in the body. While many things may trigger inflammation, the foods we choose in our diets have a profound effect on the level of inflammation in our bodies. And when chronic inflammation exists, weight gain often follows. In this chapter, we will discuss the anti-inflammatory diet, which will not only help you lose weight but also lead a much healthier life.

History of the Anti-Inflammatory Diet

When considering the anti-inflammatory diet, its history is much more recent than many of the other diets discussed in this book. In fact, it actually became popular in the last few decades. The reason the anti-inflammatory diet was a latecomer to the dieting scene relates to the fact that it is founded in recent scientific discoveries. Despite evidence supporting its use decades prior, only recently has a consensus among researchers occurred that embraced the anti-inflammatory diet's positive health effects.

The first research evidence that supported the anti-inflammatory diet was conducted by Dr. John Yudkan, a research nutritionist out of Cambridge in the late 1930s. His studies suggested that refined sugar was detrimental to one's health because of inflammatory effects. But his theory was not well accepted at the time. Instead, a focus of concern centered on saturated fats and their relationship to heart disease. This eventually led the USDA to make recommendations for eating a low fat, high carbohydrate diet. Not only did these recommendations include refined grains and sugars in the diet, but they also included processed foods and vegetable oils high in omega-6 fatty acids. Today, all of these are known to cause inflammation in the body, and many experts link these diets to our current obesity epidemic.[70]

It was not until the late 1980s that scientists began to discover that high carb diets were actually linked to weight gain and poor health. Likewise, evidence began to accumulate that many of the common food substances in most people's diet were highly inflammatory. In 1988, Dr. Art Ayers was among the first to report that refined carbohydrates, sugars, and omega-6 fatty acids triggered inflammation while also showing that fiber, vitamin C and omega-3 fatty acids were anti-inflammatory. In his blog, "Cooling Inflammation," he advocated a diet that avoided inflammation-causing foods and instead included anti-inflammation ones. His recommendations formed the foundation of the anti-inflammatory diet.[71]

What Is the Anti-Inflammatory Diet?

The anti-inflammatory diet is similar to many of the other Diet Stacking approved diets in that the food selections encouraged are naturally healthy and nutritious. But at the same time, the focus of the anti-inflammatory diet is on the inclusion of foods that reduce inflammation while avoiding those that trigger it. In doing so, you not only improve your metabolism and lose excess weight, but you enjoy greater energy and vitality. And, you also reduce your risk for developing a number of chronic illnesses that become more common with age.

In considering foods that you will want to avoid, the anti-inflammatory diet has a few broad categories that need your attention. The first category involves sugars and refined carbohydrates. These substances cause rapid rises in blood glucose levels and are known to trigger inflammation throughout the body. The second group of foods to avoid are those that have been processed. This includes processed meats and a variety of other prepackaged or preserved foods. Lastly, the anti-inflammatory diet encourages you to avoid foods with saturated or trans fats since these are also associated with chronic inflammatory responses. By avoiding these food groups, you will substantially lower the amount of inflammation in your body, which in turn, will help you lose weight and feel healthier.

At the same time, several foods can actually reduce inflammation within the body. Some foods boost anti-inflammatory prostaglandins and provide various antioxidants that keep inflammation in check. As a result, your metabolism and bodily functions improve resulting in better health and weight. In addition to fresh fruits and vegetables, which are loaded with antioxidants and nutritious substances, other anti-inflammatory foods include various spices, nuts, whole grains, and fatty fishes. Likewise, some unsaturated oils and high-protein legumes also offer benefits. Including these types of foods in your diet represents the other major component of the anti-inflammatory diet.

Why the Anti-Inflammatory Diet Works

An anti-inflammatory diet naturally strives to reduce chronic inflammation, which is linked to weight gain and poor health. But that does not mean that all types of inflammation are bad. Inflammation is actually a normal process in the body that helps us fight off infections and some cancers. During acute inflammation, your immune system becomes activated to help restore your body to its normal level of health. But sometimes, inflammation can become chronic, and instead of helping your body function better, it can make it worse. Chronic inflammation of tissues and organs can therefore undermine function leading to all types of diseases as well as weight gain.

Your diet is among one of the most important determinants of the level of chronic inflammation in your body. Certainly, managing your stress levels are important as is avoiding toxins in the environment. But the food you choose can also trigger or suppress chronic inflammation. If our diet contains pro-inflammatory foods, then blood pressure may rise, vascular disease may develop, and our metabolism may slow. Hormone systems may perform less well, and even our immune system can become exhausted, increasing the risk of infections and cancers. By reducing inflammation in the body, the anti-inflammatory diet allows your body to again achieve optimal health. And optimal health includes a healthy metabolism and a normal weight.

The Anti-Inflammatory Diet as Part of Your Stack

To understand the benefits of the anti-inflammatory diet as it pertains to both weight loss and health, it is important to know exactly which foods to include and which ones to avoid. In addition, several best practices can help you achieve the best results while on the anti-inflammatory diet. The following offers some insights in this regard to help you implement the anti-inflammatory diet effectively as part of your Diet Stack.

- Choose a variety of fresh foods, including fruits and vegetables of various colors
- Maintain portion control in addition to making wise food selections
- Drink plenty of water while avoiding sodas and sugar-sweetened beverages
- Replace refined carbs and sugars with whole grains (in moderation)

- Replace processed meats and fatty meats with fatty fish and legume proteins
- Replace saturated fats and vegetable oils with extra-virgin olive oils and unsaturated fats
- Manage your stress and invest in an active lifestyle

Using these general tips and guidelines, you can now construct your Diet Stack using the following list of foods that you will want to include and avoid as part of an anti-inflammatory diet. These food recommendations align with the best practices and will help ensure that you reduce inflammation while achieving a more ideal weight and state of health.

Anti-Inflammatory Diet Foods Allowed	Anti-Inflammatory Diet Foods to Avoid
Green leafy vegetables are particularly recommended	All refined, processed or pre-packaged foods
An array of fresh, organic fruits and vegetables in a variety of colors including tomatoes and avocados	Fruit juices that are artificially sweetened, have refined sugar, or excessively caloric
Whole grains, breads and pastas in moderation	Refined flour or bread products
Nuts and legumes including walnuts, almond, and cashews as well as these nut butters	Peanuts and peanut butters with sweeteners and/or saturated fats
Fatty fish including salmon, sardines, and herring (omega-3 fatty acids)	Fatty meats, processed meats, and all fried foods

Anti-Inflammatory Diet Foods Allowed	Anti-Inflammatory Diet Foods to Avoid
Extra-virgin olive oil and avocado oil	Margarine, vegetable oils and shortening, butters and creams
Turmeric, curcumin, ginger, and garlic encouraged	Honey, agave, and artificial sweeteners

With these insights, you can create your own anti-inflammatory meal plan. The basic rule is to select foods that have high antioxidants, detoxifying properties, and high nutrient density. At the same time, simply avoid those foods that contain potential toxins, cause rapid shifts in glucose levels, or contain fats that trigger inflammation. The following offers a sample day on an anti-inflammatory diet.

Sample Anti-Inflammatory Day

Breakfast: 2 scrambled eggs with sliced avocado and tomato

Lunch: Kale and quinoa salad

Snack: Sliced apple and 5 walnuts

Dinner: Salmon stir-fry

(Note: Full meal plans are provided in chapters 15, 16 and 17 and recipes are included in Appendix I)

The Anti-Inflammatory Diet –
The Company You Keep

As you might imagine, some of the most youthful and fit people in the world tout the anti-inflammatory diet as being essential to their wellness and physique. Two of the most well-known celebrities include Tom Brady, the New England Patriots famed quarterback, and Gisele Bundchen, his wife and international supermodel.[72] Both are committed to an anti-inflammatory diet, and the results have paid off tremendously as anyone can see. Catherine Zeta-Jones offers another example of a celebrity who recommends the anti-inflammatory diet.[73] Her seemingly timeless beauty also offers some proof of this diet's benefits.

There are many reasons why the anti-inflammatory diet represents a great choice as a diet in your Diet Stack. Certainly, its ability to reduce inflammation and the risk of chronic disease is a powerful one, but it also offers a healthy approach to weight loss and wellbeing. By following the guidelines in this chapter, you can give your body healthy nutrition while protecting it from harmful substances. This will permit your body to function at its best, and in the process, allow you to gain more energy, lose excess weight, and look your absolute best.

CHAPTER 11:

THE VEGAN DIET

Many people naturally choose vegan diets for reasons other than weight loss. Some choose vegan diets because of ethical beliefs about animal protection, while others believe vegan diets are better from an environmental perspective. And still others simply choose veganism because of the potential health benefits. But a vegan diet can also promote significant weight loss if a few best practices are kept in mind. This is one of the reasons more than a million people in the U.S. today have adopted a vegan diet as part of their lifestyle.

History of the Vegan Diet

In considering the origins of the vegan diet, the basic dietary principles align with those of vegetarians. Though early vegetarians did not necessarily avoid milk and eggs, they still chose a diet that considered the impact of their food choices on the well-being of animals. In fact, as early as 500 BCE, Greek philosopher and mathematician Pythagoras (of Pythagorean theorem fame) ate a vegetarian diet out of "benevolence" to all species. Similarly, ancient followers of Buddhism, Hinduism and Jainism also embraced a vegetarian lifestyle for the same reasons.[74] These views formed the foundation of veganism today.

While some notable individuals began objecting to dairy and eggs on ethical grounds in the nineteenth century, the term "vegan" was not coined until 1944. At that time, Donald Watson, a British woodworker, wanted to distinguish those who avoided dairy and eggs from vegetarians in general. In an effort to shorten the phrase "non-dairy vegetarians," Watson came up with the term "vegan." The name stuck, and the number of vegan diet followers has grown significantly since.[75]

Today, vegan diets are quite common with several developments encouraging many to adopt a vegan lifestyle. For one, concerns over climate change have resulted in higher rates of veganism. The industrialization of animal food production contributes significantly to greenhouse gas production, and some individuals choosing vegan diets want to do their part to reduce the impact. Likewise, this same animal processing has resulted in food products that are not necessarily the healthiest. This has provided an incentive for some people to switch to veganism. However, plenty of people also have chosen vegan diets because of the simple health and weight loss benefits that it provides. Regardless of the reasons, vegan diets have never been as popular as they are today.

What Is a Vegan Diet?

In thinking about a vegan diet, the overall concept is quite simple. Essentially, people on a vegan diet avoid all types of foods derived from animals. This naturally includes all animal meats, fish, dairy, and eggs. However, it also includes things like honey, gelatin, and whey. Why? Because these foodstuffs are also produced from animals or animal byproducts. For example, a vegan diet does not allow you to eat mayonnaise (eggs), marshmallows (gelatin), or Caesar salad dressing (anchovies). Thus, choosing a vegan diet does require greater knowledge and awareness of the foods you are eating.

One approach in eating a vegan diet is to define what is allowed. For example, fruits and vegetables are a major part of a vegan diet. Likewise, nuts, seeds, beans, and legumes are also an important part. And whole grains of all types are permitted including vegan breads, cereals and egg-free pastas. Therefore, plenty of food choices exist for people on a vegan diet. But veganism still requires a conscious effort to select healthier foods over unhealthy ones to ensure you are receiving appropriate nutrition. This is particularly important when it comes to weight loss goals.

Today, the food industry has greatly expanded food options for people who eat vegan diets. Vegan cookies, cakes, and pastries are readily available as are vegan snacks and energy bars. Likewise, meat substitutes that are vegan friendly are available with some being quite tasty. But when it comes to your well-being and to losing weight, these vegan foods may not be your best friend. Indeed, vegan diets can work very well in helping you lose weight, but understanding how vegan diets accomplish this is essential in selecting the right vegan options.

Why Vegan Diets Work

Without question, vegan diets can provide significant weight loss while also promoting better health. But this may not be the case if poor food choices are made. For example, many processed "meats" and snacks that are vegan in nature are not necessarily healthy. These can contain sugars and additives that not only add calories to your diet but also various chemicals and substances that have no nutritional value. In addition, some people swap out animal meats and dairy for higher amounts of starches and grains. As a result, they end up constantly "carb-loading," which can definitely undermine weight loss attempts.

As with any diet, making healthy food choices and watching overall calories still matter. This is certainly true for vegan diets as well. Eating too many calories even if your diet is primarily plant-based can undermine your ability to lose weight. Likewise, choosing vegan snacks and pastries will provide your body with "empty" calories void of necessary nutrients. Vegan diets help you lose weight when healthy food choices are made, which is very important to keep in mind when making a vegan diet part of your Diet Stack.

Fortunately, by making smart decisions, you can enjoy weight loss and better health on a vegan diet. When you make vegetables and fruits the major part of your vegan diet, you'll provide your body with an abundance of vitamins, minerals, and nutrients. Likewise, by making sure you get adequate protein calories from beans, tofu, and legumes, you'll be less likely to have carbohydrate cravings. And by choosing the right vitamin supplements to compliment your diet, you'll avoid some of the common pitfalls of a vegan diet.

The Vegan Diet as Part of Your Stack

If weight loss is your goal, then making good food choices while on a vegan diet is important. In addition to knowing which foods are allowed and which ones should be avoided, some other guidelines can be used to help you make good choices. If done well, a vegan diet will not only help you lose the weight you want, but will also help you achieve better health and quality of life along the way. The following are some best practices when making a vegan diet part of your Diet Stack.

- Choose nutritious, healthy options when replacing non-vegan foods with vegan options
- Include enough protein in your diet (beans, tofu and legumes are best sources)
- Limit refined carbohydrates (sugars) and avoid excessive starches (potatoes, grains)
- Monitor both portion size and calories along the way
- Consider vitamin and mineral supplements (especially B12 and iron)

Vegan diets are fairly straightforward when it comes to foods allowed and foods that should be avoided. But some may not necessarily be intuitive, especially when animal-based foods are hidden among several ingredients. The following table can be used as a guide in selecting foods that may or may not be included in your Vegan Diet Stack.

Vegan Diet Foods Allowed	Vegan Diet Foods to Avoid
Fresh vegetables of all kinds	All animal meats – beef, chicken, pork, etc.
Fresh fruits of all kinds	All fish and seafood
Nuts, nut butters, and seeds	All dairy products – milk, yogurt, cream, cheese, butter, whey
Beans and legumes	All eggs and egg products (mayonnaise)
Whole grains and cereals – wheat, rice, oats, quinoa	Honey, bee pollen
Nut milks, vegan cheeses, and yogurts – almond, coconut, rice-based	Gelatins and isinglass (used in making some wine and beer)
Tofu and minimally processed meat substitutes	Highly processed foods and those with lots of preservatives
Vegan beer and wine, all spirits	Limit vegan desserts and snacks

As indicated in the table above, just because something is "vegan" on the label doesn't mean you should necessarily include it in your diet. The vegan diet is an excellent way to lose weight and achieve better health. However, the most significant benefits are gained when fresh fruits and vegetables comprise a significant amount of the daily meal plan with adequate protein sources. With this in mind, the following provides a sample day on a Vegan diet.

Sample Vegan Diet Day

<u>Day 1</u>

    Breakfast: Avocado toast

    Lunch: Roasted cauliflower salad

    Snack: Apple with almond butter

    Dinner: Spaghetti squash with white beans and pesto

> *(Note: Full meal plans are provided in chapters 15, 16 and 17 and recipes are included in Appendix I)*

Vegan Dieting – The Company You Keep

When it comes to celebrities who embrace a vegan lifestyle, several enthusiastically promote it as a healthy way of eating. For Miley Cyrus, she chooses a vegan diet because it aligns with her values and beliefs about the ethical treatment of animals. But at the same time, she enjoys the health benefits it provides. Jessica Chastain is also an advocate for vegan diets. In addition to its ability to help her maintain an ideal weight, she boasts about the energy boost and clearer skin a vegan lifestyle provides. And Michelle Pfeiffer, who seems to be ageless, attributes her persistent beauty in part to vegan dieting as well.[76]

You may have a number of reasons why a vegan diet might appeal to you. But if weight loss is something you desire, then including a vegan diet in your Diet Stack offers some important advantages. Unlike some of the other diets, vegan diets are not as restrictive. In addition, if healthy foods are chosen, a vegan diet will likely boost your energy while also helping you feel slender and trim. By paying attention to a few important guidelines, a vegan diet offers a nutritious, healthy approach to weight loss. And it is one diet that can easily be adopted for a lifetime.

CHAPTER 12:

THE MEDITERRANEAN DIET

As one of the most popular diets in the world, the Mediterranean diet is known for its health benefits as well as for its potential in helping with weight loss. The Mediterranean diet offers a simple yet very customizable approach to losing weight, and including it in your Stack may open your eyes to a new way of life. After all, who wouldn't want to adopt a lifestyle as if living along the Mediterranean coast? The following describes what the Mediterranean diet entails and what it doesn't so you can better decide if this Diet Stacking approved option works for you.

History of the Mediterranean Diet

When it comes to the Mediterranean basin, the region has been described as the "cradle" of all civilizations. Because so many cultures originated from these areas of the world, the Mediterranean diet reflects influences that are quite diverse in nature. Not only did the ancient Greeks play a role in defining the cuisine of the region, but so did ancient Rome, Islamic cultures, Persian and Ottoman empires, and, to an extent, European nations.[77] Understanding this, the Mediterranean diet is not a diet as strictly defined as many of the other diets you might consider in your Diet Stack.

Historically speaking, the foundation of the Mediterranean diet evolved from Greek culture. The Greek word "diaita" provides the root origin for our word "diet," but in Greek, the term actually refers to a lifestyle rather than foods alone. In other words, "diet" was more about a way of living for the Greeks. Subsequently, during the peak of the Roman Empire, the Romans adopted this same perspective that the Greeks had embraced. As a result, many of the same foods that comprised most of the Greek cuisine was also part of the Roman diet. Many of the primary foods that comprise the Mediterranean diet today still reflect these influences.[78]

After the Roman dynasty, dietary choices around the Mediterranean Sea were influenced by other civilizations as well. Arab, Egyptian, and European influences played a role in creating the Mediterranean diets of the modern era. But scientific investigations in the 1980s revealed the significant health benefits that the Mediterranean diet provided. The Mediterranean diet was suddenly recognized as a means to not only lose weight and be healthy but as a way to prolong your life as well![79] These discoveries are why the Mediterranean diet is so popular today. And, at the same time, its simplicity and rich heritage make the diet quite appealing.

What Is a Mediterranean Diet?

Unlike other diets in this book, the Mediterranean diet didn't actually begin as a food diet. Because the ancient Greeks perceived food as more of a way of life, the Mediterranean diet actually focused on an active lifestyle at its core. Not only did this mean being active physically, but it also meant being socially engaged and eating meals with others.

With that in mind, you might say the Mediterranean diet is more of a holistic approach to weight loss and health!

Appreciating this aspect of the Mediterranean diet philosophy, the primary foods that made up the Mediterranean diet were bread, olive oil and wine for ancient Mediterranean civilizations. These foods are still an important part of the Mediterranean diet today with whole grains, healthy saturated oils, and unprocessed or refined breads being a major part. In addition, the Mediterranean diet also includes fresh vegetables, fruits, nuts, seeds and legumes as important parts of the diet. All of these foods, as well as natural herbs and spices, should be eaten every day. And as you can see, all of these foods are quite healthy based on what we now know about the human body.

In terms of proteins, the Mediterranean diet encourages eating fish and seafood twice a week. These foods supplement the proteins found in beans, nuts and legumes in the daily diet. However, other proteins like poultry, eggs, and dairy products should be eaten only once a week and in moderate portions. Likewise, red meats should only be eaten on rare occasions as should sweets and desserts. And unlike other diets, red wine is actually encouraged if you choose. One to two glasses a day have been a traditional part of the Mediterranean diet. Thus as a summary, the Mediterranean diet is one that is high in olive oil, legumes and vegetables and moderate to high in protein (from fish) and moderate in carbohydrates that are typical of this region of the world.

Why Mediterranean Diets Work

When it comes to Mediterranean diets, research has identified several health benefits. For example, the Mediterranean diet has been shown to reduce the risk of heart disease and some cancers. It also reduces the chance of diabetes and metabolic syndromes associated with obesity. The Mediterranean diet has even been linked to lower rates of degenerative brain disorders like dementia. As you can see, this diet has a number of health advantages that go well beyond weight loss.

But how does the Mediterranean diet work? In looking at the health benefits that it provides, a single answer doesn't exist. Instead, the Mediterranean diet promotes health and weight loss through a variety of ways. For one, the diet is naturally high in fiber. The whole grains, nuts, seeds, and vegetables provide ample fiber that can reduce cholesterol levels as well as the risk of some cancers like colon cancer. In addition, the fats in the Mediterranean diet are healthy fats. Olive oil and avocados are unsaturated fats, which provides your body with energy without increasing the risk for vascular disease and plaque. And the Mediterranean diet has tons of vitamins and nutrients from the fresh produce, fish, and seafood. These provide things like antioxidants, omega-3s, and phytochemicals that reduce inflammation and boost your memory.

Based on current science, it seems the Mediterranean diet has all the right foods for better health and wellness.[80] But how does it lower your weight? One of the important features of the Mediterranean diet is its avoidance of refined and processed foods. That means things like sugars, processed flours, preservatives and additives are eliminated from the diet. It also avoids many of the unhealthy fats that might be found in other types of oils, margarines, fatty meats and dairy. Each of these dietary components are commonly associated with weight gain. Thus, in addition to watching your calories with the goal of losing weight, the Mediterranean diet helps you avoid common foods that often sabotage your efforts.

The Mediterranean Diet as Part of Your Stack

Including the Mediterranean diet in your Diet Stack can be helpful in a number of ways. Naturally, this diet offers a health plan that provides numerous health advantages while also helping you lose weight. Likewise, it is a diet that can be easily maintained for a lifetime, and it can also be easily combined with other Diet Stacking approved diets. However, using the Mediterranean diet as a weight loss approach does require some discipline and some oversight. The following can help you achieve these goals while also making sure you follow the diet correctly.

- Choose fresh, whole foods whenever possible including vegetables, fruits and grains
- Avoid all foods that have been processed, refined, or preserved
- If you choose to drink wine, red wine is preferred and limit to 1-2 glasses a day

- Olive oil should be extra-virgin olive oil
- Be sure to also pursue an active and social lifestyle in the process
- Monitor portion size and calories to ensure weight loss

Overall, the Mediterranean diet allows you to have some significant flexibility in determining what you choose to eat. Given the fact that actual Mediterranean diets vary greatly in different regions, this only makes logical sense. But at the same time, a guide for identifying which foods should be considered and which ones should be avoided is helpful. The following can be used as such a guide in formulating your Mediterranean meal plan.

Mediterranean Diet Foods Allowed	Mediterranean Diet Foods to Avoid
Fresh fruits of all kinds including apples, bananas, pears, grapes, dates, figs and more	Processed foods or those with heavy additives or preservatives
Fresh vegetables of all kinds including kale, broccoli, spinach, onions, carrots and more	Refined oils such as soybean oil, canola oil or cottonseed oil
Nuts and seeds of all varieties	Sugar sweetened beverages or foods with added sugars
Legumes including beans, chickpeas, lentils and peas	Limit dairy and poultry to once a week
Extra virgin olive oil, avocado oil	Limit red meat to monthly portions and choose lean options

Mediterranean Diet Foods Allowed	Mediterranean Diet Foods to Avoid
Fresh fish and seafood including salmon, trout, sardines, clams, mussels and more	Trans-fats and saturated fats including margarine
Whole grain breads, cereals and pastas (in moderation)	Refined breads and flour products
Red wine up to 1-2 glasses a day if preferred	Beer, white wine, and other alcohol should be limited to rare occasions

Although I provide a detailed Mediterranean three-day meal plan in section three, using this table as a guide, you can create a meal plan based on your own food preferences and tastes. For now, here is a quick sample day on the Mediterranean diet.

Sample Mediterranean Diet Day

Breakfast: Greek frittata

Lunch: Quinoa stuffed peppers

Snack: White bean hummus and veggies

Dinner: Grilled salmon and roasted Brussels sprouts with 1 glass red wine (optional)

(Note: Full meal plans are provided in chapters 15, 16 and 17 and recipes are included in Appendix I)

Mediterranean Dieting – The Company You Keep

It's no secret that many celebrities enjoy the Mediterranean diet. For example, Penelope Cruz, whose heritage is Spanish, naturally chooses Mediterranean diet foods as part of her culture and health. But some major Hollywood stars have really shown just how effective the Mediterranean diet can be for weight loss. Specifically, John Goodman has lost nearly 100 pounds since adopting the Mediterranean diet. Also, Rachel Ray has admitted to losing two inches around the waistline by sticking to a Mediterranean diet.[81]

If you think the Mediterranean diet is a good fit for you, then including it in your Diet Stack can provide you with a way to lose weight while improving your overall wellness. This is why many opt to include this diet as part of their overall Diet Stacking strategy.

CHAPTER 13:

THE LOW-CALORIE DIET

It seems pretty intuitive that anyone can lose weight by simply cutting the calories in their diet. In fact, you have likely tried doing this throughout your life for one reason or another. Perhaps you had a big event or vacation, and you wanted to look your best. Or maybe you were trying to jumpstart a new, healthier lifestyle. In either case, you naturally appreciated that a lower calorie diet could help you lose weight. And you were right!

In terms of Diet Stacking the low-calorie diet represents a healthy, low-calorie approach to weight loss that can be adjusted and maintained over time if you desire. When done correctly and for only short bursts (as is the case with Diet Stacking) the low-calorie diet can offer rapid weight loss and other health benefits. This makes the low-calorie diet a popular option for those trying to lose weight while paying attention to overall wellness.

History of the Low-Calorie Diet

When considering the history of the low-calorie diet, it seems only fitting to discuss when the term "calorie" was first used. Interestingly, it wasn't until the mid-19th century that the word calorie was used in physics' language to describe energy. And it wasn't related to food consumption until 1887 when W.O. Atwater published an article in *Century* magazine. From that time on, Americans began to compare calories in food to their body weight, and the low-calorie diet became a common practice.

But reducing calories to lose weight is not exactly the same as the low-calorie diet described for your Diet Stack. The version of the low-calorie diet that is utilized for the purpose of Diet Stacking stems from research done out of the United Kingdom. The research, published in 2016 from Newcastle University, described 30 overweight or obese diabetic individuals' experience on a low carbohydrate, very low-calorie diet for 8 weeks. The individuals in the study lost an average of 30 pounds and kept the weight off for 6 months. In addition, nearly half were able to reverse their diabetes![82]

The calorie restriction in the research study was less than 700 calories a day, but the popular version of the low-calorie diet today allows 800 calories. Dr. Michael Mosely, a British physician demonstrated how this type of diet can be very effective for long term weight loss in thousands of people.[83] And you don't have to be obese or diabetic to enjoy the many benefits of the low-calorie diet approach.

What Is the Low-Calorie Diet?

The low-calorie diet for the purposes of Diet Stacking is more than a reduced calorie meal plan. In fact, it combines features of some of the other diets described in this book including the Mediterranean diet and the low carb diet. The bottom line is you must limit your calories to 800 calories a day during your three-day Diet Stack. In doing so, you are encouraged to select specific foods that offer better health and wellness as well as weight loss. In this way, you will be much more likely to see great results not only on the scales but also in the way you feel.

The low-calorie diet encourages you to eat fresh vegetables, lean protein and healthy oils, nuts and seeds (in moderation). It also encourages eating fish and seafood for your protein while limiting red meats. In terms of dairy, hard cheeses and unsweetened yogurts can be included but should be eaten in moderation. Choosing these foods and keeping your calories to 800 calories a day defines the low-calorie diet in your Stack. As you can see, it has many features of both the Mediterranean diet and low-carb diet while adding an additional twist on the number of daily calories you can have.

Why Low-Calorie Diets Work

It's no big secret why a low-calorie diet works in promoting weight loss. Fewer calories in your diet results in more stored calories being burned. And this results in weight loss over time. But the low-calorie diet works in several different ways to not only help boost weight loss but to also make you healthier. In addition to its ability to help you lose weight quickly, the low-calorie diet also reduces your risks for heart disease, stroke, and diabetes. And it has been shown to improve your ability to sleep while making you feel more energetic and active.[84]

First, by restricting your calories to 800 a day, you immediately shift your body's metabolism. Instead of only burning food calories from your diet for energy, you start burning calories from stored fats. This shift is a big reason people on a low-calorie diet see weight loss results so quickly! But at the same time, the low-calorie diet lets you still include fats in your diet. This helps deter some of the cravings and hunger that can naturally come with a low-calorie approach. And as long as you stick to the 800 calories a day you can also include some indulgences along the way that will help ensure you don't feel deprived.

The Low-Calorie Diet as Part of Your Stack

The low-calorie diet requires some considerations. During your three-day low calorie diet, you will certainly experience hunger simply because of the reduction in calories. But specific foods can help deter this to an extent. And remember your low-calorie Stack only lasts three days. This short duration will help you stay motivated. Likewise, because your body will be shifting toward fat metabolism, hydration is very important. The following provides some recommendations that might help you with your Low-Calorie Diet Stack.

- Choose foods high in fiber which will improve satiety and health effects
- Hydrate well with plenty of water throughout the Diet Stack period

- For the three-day period, replace red meat with fish, seafood or lean poultry
- Consider hot soups and beverages as these also reduce hunger
- Fresh, whole foods should be chosen with avoidance of processed or refined foods

Low-calorie diet foods allowed are comparable to those of the Mediterranean diet but with greater attention to how many carbohydrates and calories you eat (<800 calories). In this regard, fruits should be monitored closely since they have higher sugar levels and calories. Likewise, starchy vegetables are not as good of a choice as leafy or fibrous vegetables due to high carbohydrate content and higher calorie count. With these additional thoughts in mind, the following provides a guide to foods you may consider or avoid as part of your Low-Calorie Diet Stack.

Low-Calorie Diet Foods Allowed	Low-Calorie Diet Foods to Avoid
Fresh fruits allowed but should be limited due to high sugar content and calories	Processed foods or those with heavy additives or preservatives
Fresh vegetables of all kinds including kale, broccoli, spinach, onions, carrots and more	Refined oils such as soybean oil, canola oil or cottonseed oil
Nuts and seeds of all varieties (in moderation)	Sugar-sweetened beverages or foods with added sugars

Low-Calorie Diet Foods Allowed	Low-Calorie Diet Foods to Avoid
Legumes such as beans, chickpeas, and lentils permitted but should be limited in portions	Most dairy products
Extra-virgin olive oil, avocado oil (in moderation)	Trans-fats and saturated fats including margarine
Fresh fish and seafood including salmon, trout, sardines, clams, mussels and more	Red meat and pork
Whole grain breads, cereals and pastas permitted but in very limited portions	Refined breads and flour products
Eggs and lean poultry	All alcohol

For the purposes of the three-day Diet Stack, the recommended low-calorie diet should stick to the 800-calorie daily restrictions and the allowed foods outlined above. However, if you decide at a later time to adopt the low-calorie diet long-term, other options exist. For example, the 5:2 diet, promoted by Dr. Michael Mosley, suggests restricting your calories twice a week and eating normally for five days.[85] This approach also provides weight and health benefits, but the rate of weight loss is more gradual. However, for your Diet Stack, you should stick to 800 calories a day for your three-day stack. In section three you will get a detailed day-by-day low calorie meal plan. For now, lets check out a simple low calorie day.

Sample Low-Calorie Diet Day

Breakfast: Vegetable omelet

Lunch: Kale, pear and pecan salad

Dinner: Chicken and vegetable soup

(Note: Full meal plans are provided in chapters 15, 16 and 17 and recipes are included in Appendix I)

Low-Calorie Dieting – The Company You Keep

The Low-Calorie Diet Stack is an excellent choice when it comes to rapid weight loss. The calorie restriction, when performed in a healthy manner, enables you to shed pounds quickly while also giving your body the nutrients it needs. Several celebrities have turned to such a low-calorie diet when rapid weight loss has been needed for various acting roles. For example, both Mila Kunis and Natalie Portman lost double-digits in a short time on low-calorie diets when filming the *Black Swan*. Likewise, Anne Hathaway has done the same during some of her films including *Les Misérables*.[86]

Of course, the low-calorie diet is not one that can be sustained indefinitely, but it's a great option when included for just three days as part of your Stack. If you choose to continue this diet after your Diet Stacking has been completed, a low-calorie diet with more liberal amounts of total calories per day could be used until you reach a healthy weight. The low-calorie diet as part of your stack offers great weight loss potential when included in your overall Diet Stack.

SECTION III:
FINDING YOUR STACK

CHAPTER 14:
GETTING STARTED

It's a commonly described statistic. Roughly, nine out of every 10 people fail at dieting. Not only do most diets fail, but people often get discouraged and fall into a cycle of "yo-yo" dieting and end up weighing more than they did when they started. While yo-yo dieting is a real thing for many, and while many diets can fail, this does not have to be the norm. In fact, research has revealed some very interesting findings when it comes to diets and keeping the weight off.

For nearly a quarter of a century, researchers at Brown University have been tracking individuals across the nation who had dieting success. Those in the registry were required to have lost at least 30 pounds and have kept the weight off for more than a year. Today, more than 10,000 people are on the registry with an average weight loss of 66 pounds per person. This clearly shows that dieting is not certain to fail but instead can actually provide great results. But then again, the devil's in the details.[87]

Among the thousands who successfully lost weight, about half followed their own unique dieting style while the other half followed structured diets. In addition, the majority had to try more than one diet before succeeding. This coincides with other research that shows one diet does not work for everyone. Just as each of us are unique in many ways, the type of diet that will help us lose weight is very individualized.[88] This is why some people struggle to stay on a specific diet while others may be successful on it. Diet Stacking is not a one-diet-fits-all program. In fact, Diet Stacking uses this knowledge to develop a "diet stack" that works best for you.

Despite the different dieting strategies used by the registry participants, several best practices were identified. From exercise to specific behaviors, key activities increased the odds that a diet would result in weight loss success. Below are ten specific things you will want to consider when starting your Diet Stack. These tips can help get you started on the right foot.

Diet Stacking Tip #1 –
Review Your Diet Stack Options

Before you can determine how to best construct your Stack, you naturally need to know which Diet Stacking approved diets are most attractive to you. As noted, a diet that works for one person may not be very effective for another. And certainly, a diet that sounds challenging and unappealing is not likely to keep you motivated and inspired. Therefore, spend a little time and get to know each of the Diet Stacking options available to you.

Be honest with yourself about which diets sound reasonable and which ones are right for you based on your preferences and lifestyle. And don't concern yourself with which ones you think will be the fastest in providing positive results. The Diet Stacks outlined in the next chapter are designed for long-term weight loss and better health. Doing a little homework, and adopting a long-range view, can go a long way in helping you successfully achieve your weight loss goals.

Diet Stacking Tip #2 –
Choose Your Diet Stack Timeline

Just as the Diet Stacking approved diets you choose offer unique dieting experiences to meet your specific needs, the duration of your Diet Stack does as well. As a reminder, a three-Stack lasts for nine days (three days for each diet in the Stack) while the 5-Stack and the 7-Stack last 15 and 21 days respectively. You might prefer a smaller number of diets over a shorter period of time. Or alternatively, you may prefer a larger number of diets in your Stack in which case you could choose to develop your own stack. Depending on your life situation and taste, the duration of your Diet Stack and the diets you choose may vary.

Diet Stacking Tip #3 –
Create Your Diet Stack Shopping List

As you might imagine, changing your diet means you might need to clean out your refrigerator and kitchen cabinets. And it means shopping for foods that align with the Stack you select. Naturally, you will not shop for the entire duration of your Diet Stack program, but it does pay to get organized ahead of time. As a result, tip #3 encourages you to plan ahead and create a shopping list for your Diet Stack program in advance.

By creating your shopping list in advance, you will be able to eliminate some of the stress that might occur with any new diet. You will be better able to focus on eating well and being positive about the changes you are making rather than trying to figure out what you need from the store each day. Though this might not seem like a major issue, planning your shopping needs ahead of time removes one obstacle that might sabotage your success. Therefore, determine what grocery items you need prior to starting your Stack so you have one less thing to think about.

Diet Stacking Tip #4 –
Prepare Your Meals and Snacks in Advance

There are plenty of times when convenience rules. Perhaps, you overslept for work, or maybe you are running late for an appointment. Sometimes, you may not be in the mood to cook. But in each of these instances, grabbing something "quick" to eat at a restaurant, drive-through, or a convenience store can be quite tempting. When these situations occur, the chance we will choose less healthy food choices becomes a real possibility.

But when you're prepared, grabbing a healthy meal or snack is easy. Simply having healthy options available instead of unhealthy ones reduces the chance for slip-ups. At the same time, being prepared also reduces your level of stress, which can also be a trigger for choosing less healthy foods. Without question, you won't be able to prepare all your meals in advance. Similarly, there will be times where convenience is a must. But preparing your meals or snacks ahead of time greatly increases your chances of sticking to your Stack, which increases the odds of having great results.

Diet Stacking Tip #5 –
Keep a Food Journal

One of the best-kept secrets in achieving your weight loss goals involves keeping a food journal. A food journal not only helps you log what specific foods you ate and their total calories, carbs, fats and proteins, but it can also be used to help you follow your emotions, challenges, and "wins." Emotional triggers can often cause you to stray from your diet plan, and by keeping a food journal, you will be better able to identify moods and feelings that might be a problem. Also, a food journal helps you record your daily improvements, which can serve as a source for ongoing motivation. A food journal can thus provide a wealth of information and insights.

In addition to these advantages, a food journal also helps you be accountable to your plan and goals. It becomes easy to see when you go astray, and as a result, you are better able to get back on track quickly. For Diet Stacking, a food journal has additional benefits as well. Because you will be cycling through a number of Diet Stacking approved diets, a food journal will help you identify the diets that were most effective and enjoyable for you. This can be extremely helpful should you choose to develop a custom Stack in the future.

Diet Stacking Tip #6 –
Drink Plenty of Water and Stay Hydrated

While many people appreciate the health benefits of staying well hydrated, not as many associate drinking plenty of water with weight loss. When our bodies are well hydrated, all of our body's cells are able to function better. This means cells are better able to respond to insulin, use glucose, and eliminate toxins. And proper hydration improves your metabolism. Each of these things help you to lose weight more efficiently.

In addition to these benefits, being well hydrated is associated with higher energy levels and a sense of wellbeing. As a result, you will be better able to manage stress and stick to a meal plan that aligns well with your goals. Lastly, choosing to drink water with your meals reduces some of the beverages that might undermine your success. Sodas, sweetened tea, caffeinated drinks, and alcoholic beverages are linked to weight gain and health issues. Therefore, choosing to drink plenty of water and maintain proper hydration simply makes good sense in helping you achieve success. Find drinking water boring? Download my free 27 Detox Water Recipes https://dawnastone.com/detox-water-recipes

These delicious water recipes will keep it interesting and help you stay hydrated!

Diet Stacking Tip #7 –
Fill Up on Fibrous Vegetables

When striving to lose weight, nearly every diet will result in some degree of hunger, especially at first. Therefore, choosing healthy foods that help "fill you up" can reduce these uncomfortable sensations and increase your chances of sticking to your diet. Fiber is excellent in this regard because fiber itself is not absorbed into your body. Instead, fiber stays in your digestive tract and helps not only improve bowel function but also bowel health. And, it is rather filling, reducing your hunger sensations.

While fiber can be obtained from whole grains, not all Diet Stack diets encourage an ample amount of this food group. However, many whole, organic, fresh vegetables have tons of fiber. Fibrous vegetables, like broccoli, Brussels sprouts, cauliflower, and others, can ease your hunger while also enhancing wellness. By filling up on fibrous vegetables, you enjoy the weight loss benefits of Diet Stacking while minimizing some of the normal struggles many have when dieting.

Diet Stacking Tip #8 –
Create a Positive Environment for Change

Diet Stacking is a great way to achieve your weight loss goals. But lasting change often requires a little extra effort to help ensure you get the results you want. With that in mind, creating a positive environment around you is strongly encouraged when pursuing any lifestyle and dietary change. What's a positive environment? For one, it means adopting a positive attitude. Speak positively about the changes you are making. Celebrate your successes. And certainly, surround yourself with positive, supportive individuals who can help keep you "up" when the going gets tough.

In addition to seeing yourself in a positive light and using positive language, a strong support network offers many advantages. Naturally, telling others about your goals and plans makes you more accountable. But at the same time, friends and family can help provide great motivation and encouragement. Support can also help you problem-solve more effectively when you are struggling with specific obstacles, and friends and family can help you avoid tricky situations. Creating a positive vibe while on your Stack will certainly be much more enjoyable and help you be more successful.

Diet Stacking Tip #9 –
Replace Unhealthy Habits with Healthy Ones

Habits can be pretty tough to break. Cravings between meals can be really challenging when starting a new diet. And suppressing those late-night munchies when all the food on television looks so delicious can really be difficult. It's important to appreciate that these unhealthy habits are not simply going to evaporate into thin air just because you have decided to lose some weight. Therefore, being proactive and taking matters into your own hands is essential.

The goal is to replace these unhealthy habits with healthy ones. For example, many of the Diet Stacking approved diets allow healthy foods like apples that can be very filling and satisfying. This can be used to replace some of your prior unhealthy snacking choices. Or you might try some herbal tea as an alternative to help distract you from your cravings. Some people have even found a 15-minute walk is enough to deter these unwanted behaviors. What works for you will be highly individualized, but replacing bad habits with new healthy ones can help you immensely in your weight loss pursuit.

Diet Stacking #10 –
Incorporate Exercise into Your Routine

It's no surprise that exercise can help you lose weight. After all, the more calories your burn, the more likely you are to lose weight. But were you aware that exercise also helps you diet as well? Regular exercise is a great way to boost your metabolism and to improve your circulation. Particularly with aerobic forms of exercise like walking, jogging and cycling, your body's cells function better as access to oxygen and circulation improves. As a result, your metabolism will increase, allowing your Diet Stack to be more effective.

In addition to these benefits, exercise is also a great appetite suppressant. That means you will be less likely to feel hungry when physically active, especially during those in-between meal times. And exercise improves your ability to sleep while also reducing stress. A good night's rest and better coping skills naturally improve your ability to stick to any diet. Therefore, adding a regular exercise program to your Diet Stacking program significantly boosts your chances of reaching your weight loss goals.

Are You Ready to Stack?

With these ten Diet Stacking tips, you are now ready to begin your own personal Diet Stacking program. Following the tips will give you the best chance of reaching your weight loss goals while pursuing a healthier diet and lifestyle in the process. And because Diet Stacking disrupts the typical diet process, it increases your motivation making it more likely that you will reach your goals.

In the next few chapters, we will explore the different Diet Stacking programs, which range from a 3-Stack to a 7-Stack. In each of these chapters, detailed and easy-to-follow Diet Stacking meal plans will be provided as well as some strategies you might consider when customizing your own Diet Stack. By combining the ten tips outlined in this chapter with the information in the subsequent chapters, you will be best able to construct the perfect Diet Stack for you. So, let's get started! It's time to Stack!

CHAPTER 15:

THE SIMPLE STACK

The first of three Diet Stacking options is the Simple Stack or 3-Stack. Why is it called the Simple Stack? Because the Simple Stack only lasts nine days and involves just three of the Diet Stack approved diets previously described. The Simple Stack allows you to quickly appreciate how Diet Stacking works and the benefits it can provide in a relatively short time period. Likewise, the Simple Stack lets you sample some of the Diet Stacking approved diets over a short period of time without a longer-term commitment.

When choosing which Diet Stacking approved diets to include in your Simple Stack, you can select any of the ten Diet Stacking approved diets outlined in Section Two. It is worth noting, however, one of the main benefits of Diet Stacking is prolonged motivation and this works best when the diets you select are not too similar. That is, they are different enough to peak motivation and to re-energize you as you start your next stack. Because the Simple Stack only involves three diets, the diets you choose to stack are extremely important. In addition, as highlighted in the *Getting Started* chapter, you might consider practical issues such as lifestyle, food likes and dislikes, etc.

Although you may combine any three Diet Stacking approved diets you like in a Simple Stack, the Stack that I have found to be quite effective is provided below. For first-time Diet Stackers and those who want to lose some weight quickly, this Simple Stack has great potential for positive results. Because of this, it is my "go-to" Simple Stack and I hope you will give it a try.

The Recommended Simple Stack (total of nine days)
- The Intermittent Fasting Diet (Days 1, 2 and 3)
- The Ketogenic Diet (Days 4, 5 and 6)
- The Vegan Diet (Days 7, 8 and 9)

This combination has some rationale behind its recommendation as a Simple Stack. By starting with the intermittent fasting diet, you provide your body the opportunity to eliminate existing toxins while promoting weight loss through better glucose metabolism. This is then followed by the ketogenic diet, which provides ample proteins after fasting, yet it prevents a rapid "reloading" of carbs back into your system. Finally, the vegan diet allows healthy carbs to be introduced along with healthy fruits and vegetables. As a result, this recommendation for a Simple Stack promotes weight loss quickly while also promoting wellness without being too "abrupt."

Of course, you may choose any three Diet Stacking approved diets when creating your own Simple Stack. But sometimes, just having a recommendation can make the decision easier or better guide the diets you select. If you choose to use the Simple Stack option provided here, a detailed nine-day meal plan is provided below. This can help you get off to a great start and best achieve the diet goals you want. The recipes for the Simple Stack Meal Plan can be found in Appendix I.

SIMPLE STACK MEAL PLAN SAMPLE

The Intermittent Fasting Diet (Days 1, 2 and 3)

Reminder: For the purposes of your Stack, intermittent fasting is defined as two fasting days and one non-fasting day. Days one and three are fasting days and should include 500-800 calories based on your activity level (as outlined in Chapter 4). Day two is a non-fasting day. You choose your foods and your calorie level on this day but remember to try and eat a "normal" day's worth of calories and try not to over compensate for your fasting days.

Day 1 (Fasting)

Breakfast: Skip breakfast (black coffee, water, tea or sparkling water until noon)

Lunch: Garden salad with grilled chicken (page 206)

Dinner: Chicken and vegetable soup (page 201)

Day 2 (Non-Fasting)

Although this is your "non-fasting" day, I would suggest you stick to the following non-fasting sample meal plan.

Breakfast: Overnight oats with berries (page 192)

Snack: Apple and almond butter (page 236)

Lunch: Four-bean salad (page 204)

Dinner: Grilled halibut with tomato, avocado and mango salsa (page 209)

<u>Day 3 (Fasting)</u>

Breakfast: Skip breakfast (black coffee, water, tea or sparkling water until noon)

Lunch: Roasted cauliflower and spinach salad (page 218)

Dinner: Chicken and vegetable soup (leftover from day one) (page 201)

The Ketogenic Diet (Days 4, 5 and 6)

Reminder: A ketogenic diet is essentially a diet that significantly restricts the amount of carbohydrates you eat each day while increasing fats and consuming moderate protein. Fat consumption should be focused on healthy fats like nuts, seeds, avocado, olive oil, fatty fish and some high-fat dairy (in moderation).

<u>Day 4</u>

Breakfast: Vegetable omelet, 2 slices bacon and 1/4 avocado, sliced (page 195)

Lunch: Greek salad with grilled chicken (page 208)

Snack: 10-15 almonds

Dinner: Salmon and bell pepper stir-fry (page 219)

Day 5

Breakfast: Baked egg and avocado (page 186)

Lunch: BLT lettuce wraps (page 200)

Snack: 1oz hard cheese of your choice

Dinner: Almond-crusted chicken (page 198) with steamed asparagus (page 229)

Day 6

Breakfast: Spinach and bacon frittata (page 193)

Lunch: Avocado, tomato and feta salad (page 199)

Snack: 8 oz full fat sugar-free yogurt

Dinner: Filet mignon and arugula salad (page 203)

The Vegan Diet (Days 7, 8 and 9)

Reminder: A vegan diet avoids all types of foods derived from animals. This naturally includes all animal meats, fish, dairy, and eggs. However, it also includes things like honey, gelatin, and whey. The diet is heavy in vegetables, fresh fruit, nuts, seeds and legumes.

Day 7

Breakfast: Berry protein smoothie with vegan protein powder (page 187)

Lunch: Kale and quinoa salad (page 212)

Snack: Homemade trail mix (page 237)

Dinner: Vegetarian chili (page 224)

Day 8

Breakfast: Overnight oats with berries (page 192)

Lunch: Vegetarian chili (leftover from night before) (page 224)

Snack: Apple and almond butter (page 236)

Dinner: Quinoa and chickpea salad (page 215)

Day 9

Breakfast: Blueberry chia pudding (page 188)

Lunch: Roasted cauliflower and spinach salad (page 218)

Snack: 10-15 almonds

Dinner: Spaghetti squash with fresh herbs (page 222)

Keeping It Simple

The Simple Stack is a great Diet Stack for beginners, those wanting to lose some pounds quickly, or for those who simply want to jumpstart their diet and get back into a healthy way of life. Remember, the detailed meal plan is designed to help you plan your stack. I wanted to make it as easy as possible for you to get started and to provide you with a 3-Stack that I know works! It is up to you whether you choose to follow the plan as provided or if you want to choose your own meals/recipes. As long as you follow the rules for each diet in the stack, you have the freedom to select your meals.

In addition, if you find it difficult to cook every meal, feel free to use the recipes more than once. That is, make extra for dinner and have it again the next day. I tend to do this when I make soup or chili. I'll make a big batch of chicken vegetable soup and have it two or three days in a row—sometimes for lunch and sometimes for dinner. If you selected the Simple Stack, you should feel ready to get started. You can do it!

CHAPTER 16:

THE WEIGHT LOSS STACK

While the Simple Stack offers a fast way to sample Diet Stacking and jumpstart your weight loss efforts, the Weight Loss Stack is designed for a slightly longer period of time and to promote even more weight loss. Also known as the 5-Stack, the Weight Loss Stack combines five different Diet Stacking approved diets over 15 days. Each Diet is followed for three days until you have cycled through all five diets in your Stack. As you can see, the Weight Loss Stack allows you more time, greater weight loss and more variety.

As mentioned in other parts of the book, Diet Stacking is not meant to be a "quick-fix" to achieving your weight loss goals. Instead, Diet Stacking allows you to adopt a long-term strategy to achieving the weight you desire and help improve your health in the process. Of course, that does not mean you shouldn't see immediate results, and this is especially true for the Weight Loss Stack. During the 15 days on the Weight Loss Stack, you should expect to lose five to 10 pounds depending on the weight at which you are starting. In addition to sampling several Diet Stacking approved diets, you should also receive positive results for your efforts with the Weight Loss Stack, and this will naturally help you stay motivated and on track to reaching your goals.

As always, feel free to customize your own personal Weight Loss Stack with the Diet Stacking approved diets you believe best suit you. However, the following Weight Loss Stack offers a suggestion for the five diets you might want to consider. For my own personal favorite Weight Loss Stack, I have found this combination of diets offers rapid weight loss. Despite it lasting slightly more than two weeks, this Weight Loss Stack recommendation is intense enough to help you lose weight fairly quickly without being overly complicated. My 5-stack weight loss combination is as follows:

Weight Loss Stack (Total of 15 days)

- The Intermittent Fasting Diet (Days 1, 2 and 3)
- The Ketogenic Diet (Days 4, 5 and 6)
- The Vegan Diet (Days 7, 8 and 9)
- The Mediterranean Diet (Days 10, 11 and 12)
- The Low-Calorie Diet (Days 13, 14 and 15)

As you can appreciate, the first three diets in the Weight Loss Stack reflect the same diets recommended for the Simple Stack. This combination of Diet Stacking approved diets remains an effective weight-loss strategy in this program just as it did for the Simple Stack. But because the Weight Loss Stack extends your dieting period by another six days, the Mediterranean diet and the low-calorie diet are also included. These are also effective diets that offer rapid weight loss and help you achieve your health goals quickly.

In addition, the Mediterranean diet offers a smooth transition between the vegan diet and the low-calorie diet. Like all Diet Stack diets, fresh, organic, whole foods are encouraged, and each of the five diets in this recommended Weight Loss Stack facilitate such choices. At the same time, grocery shopping for this combination of diets is not difficult if planned ahead of time. Many of the same foods can be used in all of the diets recommended in the Weight Loss Stack.

While other excellent diet combinations exist in constructing your Weight Loss Stack, the following offers a detailed meal plan should you choose to use the recommended Weight Loss Stack described. The recipes for the Weight Loss Stack Meal Plan can be found in Appendix I.

WEIGHT LOSS STACK MEAL PLAN SAMPLE

The Intermittent Fasting Diet (Days 1, 2 and 3)

Reminder: For the purposes of your Stack, intermittent fasting is defined as two fasting days and one non-fasting day. Days one and three are fasting days and should include 500-800 calories based on your activity level (as outlined in Chapter 4). Day two is a non-fasting day. You choose your foods and your calorie level on this day but remember to try and eat a "normal" day's worth of calories and try not to over compensate for your fasting days.

Day 1 (Fasting)

Breakfast: Skip breakfast (black coffee, water, tea or sparkling water until noon)

Lunch: Garden salad with grilled chicken (page 206)

Dinner: Chicken and vegetable soup (page 201)

Day 2 (Non-Fasting)

Although this is your "non-fasting" day, I would suggest you stick to the following non-fasting sample meal plan.

Breakfast: Overnight oats with berries (page 192)

Snack: Apple and almond butter (page 236)

Lunch: Four-bean salad (page 204)

Dinner: Grilled halibut with tomato, avocado and mango salsa (page 209)

Day 3 (Fasting)

Breakfast: Skip breakfast (black coffee, water, tea or sparkling water until noon)

Lunch: Roasted cauliflower and spinach salad (page 218)

Dinner: Chicken and vegetable soup (leftover from day one) (page 201)

The Ketogenic Diet (Days 4, 5 and 6)

Reminder: A ketogenic diet is essentially a diet that significantly restricts the amount of carbohydrates you eat each day while increasing fats and consuming moderate protein. Fat consumption should be focused on healthy fats like nuts, seeds, avocado, olive oil, fatty fish and some high-fat dairy (in moderation).

Day 4

Breakfast: Vegetable omelet, 2 slices bacon and 1/4 avocado, sliced (page 195)

Lunch: Greek salad with grilled chicken (page 208)

Snack: 10-15 almonds

Dinner: Salmon and bell pepper stir-fry (page 219)

Day 5

Breakfast: Baked egg and avocado (page 186)

Lunch: BLT lettuce wraps (page 200)

Snack: 1oz hard cheese of your choice

Dinner: Almond-crusted chicken (page 198) with steamed asparagus (page 229)

Day 6

Breakfast: Spinach and bacon frittata (page 193)

Lunch: Avocado, tomato and feta salad (page 199)

Snack: 8oz full fat sugar-free yogurt

Dinner: Filet mignon and arugula salad (page 203)

The Vegan Diet (Days 7, 8 and 9)

Reminder: A vegan diet avoids all types of foods derived from animals. This naturally includes all animal meats, fish, dairy, and eggs. However, it also includes things like honey, gelatin, and whey. The diet is heavy in vegetables, fresh fruit, nuts, seeds and legumes.

Day 7

Breakfast: Berry protein smoothie with vegan protein powder (page 187)

Lunch: Kale and quinoa salad (page 212)

Snack: Homemade trail mix (page 237)

Dinner: Vegetarian chili (page 224)

Day 8

Breakfast: Overnight oats with berries (page 192)

Lunch: Vegetarian chili (leftover from night before) (page 224)

Snack: Apple and almond butter (page 236)

Dinner: Quinoa and chickpea salad (page 215)

Day 9

Breakfast: Blueberry chia pudding (page 188)

Lunch: Roasted cauliflower and spinach salad (page 218)

Snack: 10-15 almonds

Dinner: Spaghetti squash with fresh herbs (page 222)

The Mediterranean Diet (Days 10, 11 and 12)

Reminder: The primary foods that make up the Mediterranean diet are fresh vegetables, fish, other seafood, whole grains, healthy oils, unprocessed or un-refined breads, nuts, seeds, legumes, some fruit (in moderation), olive oil and wine. In addition, natural herbs and spices are used to enhance the flavor of the meal. Other proteins like poultry, eggs, and dairy products should be eaten only once a week and in moderate portions. Likewise, red meats should only be eaten on rare occasions, as should sweets and desserts. And unlike other diets, red wine is actually encouraged if you choose.

Day 10

> Breakfast: Avocado toast (page 185)
>
> Snack: Apple and almond butter (page 236)
>
> Lunch: Avocado, tomato and feta salad (page 199)
>
> Dinner: Shrimp stir-fry (page 220)

Day 11

> Breakfast: Greek yogurt with fresh berries (page 192)
>
> Lunch: Spinach salad with strawberries and walnuts (page 223)
>
> Snack: 10-15 almonds
>
> Dinner: Quinoa stuffed peppers (page 216)

Day 12

Breakfast: Greek frittata (page 191)

Lunch: Quinoa stuffed peppers (left over from night before) (page 216)

Snack: White bean hummus and veggies (page 238)

Dinner: Ginger salmon (page 207) and roasted Brussels sprouts (page 227)

The Low-Calorie Diet (Days 13, 14 and 15)

Reminder: For your Stack, a low-calorie diet is defined as no more than 800 calories a day. (Remember, your stack only lasts three days!) By restricting your calories, instead of only burning food calories from your diet for energy, you start burning calories from stored fats—helping you lose weight fast. During your low-calorie Stack choose foods high in fiber, hydrate well, replace red meat with fish, seafood or lean poultry, consider hot soups and beverages as these also reduce hunger and choose fresh, whole foods rather than processed or refined foods.

Day 13

Breakfast: Vegetable omelet (page 195)

Lunch: Kale, pear and pecan salad (page 214)

Dinner: Chicken and vegetable soup (page 201)

Day 14

Breakfast: Overnight oats with berries (page 192)

Lunch: Chicken and vegetable soup (left over from the night before) (page 201)

Dinner: Spinach salad with strawberries and walnuts (page 223)

Day 15

Breakfast: Green veggie juice (page 190)

Lunch: Quinoa and chickpea salad (page 215)

Dinner: Grilled herb chicken (page 210) with steamed broccoli (page 230)

Ready to Shed Some Pounds?

The Weight Loss Stack is ideal for those who want to lose weight relatively quickly and sample a number of excellent Diet Stacking approved options. While the Weight Loss Stack is great for beginners, especially if choosing the recommended Weight Loss Stack combination outlined, it is also fantastic for anyone wanting to lose up to 10 pounds in a relatively short time frame. This is why the Weight Loss Stack is the most popular Diet Stack!

CHAPTER 17:

THE EXTREME STACK

The next Diet Stack offered is the Extreme Stack, which lets you take your Diet Stacking to the max! Also known as the 7-Stack, the Extreme Stack invites you to combine seven Diet Stacking approved diets for three weeks with each diet lasting three days. As you might imagine, this allows you to experience a variety of Diet Stacking approved diets while adhering to a strict weight loss regimen that is certain to produce results.

In describing the Extreme Stack, I often refer to this Diet Stack as the 21-Day Diet Stacking Challenge. Given its duration and the number of Diet Stacking approved diets involved, the Extreme Stack is more challenging than other short Diet Stacking options. But the Extreme Stack can be expected to help you lose as much as 10 to 15 pounds in a 21-day period. In addition, the Extreme Stack lets you sample a much larger number of dieting styles, and this can help keep your motivation at its peak.

While the Extreme Stack may be more challenging if you are just beginning to Diet Stack, it is certainly not impossible. However, the Extreme Stack does require more planning and organizing to ensure better success. This includes grocery shopping, meal planning, and accommo-dating the transitions between diets along the way. But if weight loss is your goal, the Extreme Stack is a great choice.

The following is the recommended program for the Extreme Stack.

Extreme Stack (Total of 21 days)

- The Intermittent Fasting Diet (Days 1, 2 and 3)
- The Ketogenic Diet (Days 4, 5 and 6)
- The Vegan Diet (Days 7, 8 and 9)
- The Mediterranean Diet (Days 10, 11 and 12)
- The Low-Calorie Diet (Days 13, 14 and 15)
- The Paleo Diet (Days 16, 17 and 18)
- The Elimination Diet (Days 19, 20 and 21)

The recommended Extreme Stack incorporates the Simple Stack and Weight Loss Stack. In addition, the Extreme Stack adds the Paleo diet and the elimination diet to complete the 21-day Diet Stacking program.

Both the Paleo diet and the elimination diet offer great potential for additional weight loss, and they both also further adopt a dietary approach that is natural and healthy while avoiding processed, preserved, or highly caloric foods. This is why they have been included as part of the Extreme Stack. In addition, both can further enhance your chances of weight loss success and wellness. As always, you are welcome to combine any of the Diet Stacking approved diets into an Extreme Stack based on personal needs and preferences. But as part of the recommended regimen cited, the following offers a detailed Extreme Stack meal plan that you can follow and is proven to work. The recipes for the Extreme Stack Meal Plan can be found in Appendix I.

EXTREME STACK MEAL PLAN SAMPLE

The Intermittent Fasting Diet (Days 1, 2 and 3)

Reminder: For the purposes of your Stack, intermittent fasting is defined as two fasting days and one non-fasting day. Days one and three are fasting days and should include 500-800 calories based on your activity level (as outlined in Chapter 4). Day two is a non-fasting day. You choose your foods and your calorie level on this day but remember to try and eat a "normal" day's worth of calories and try not to over compensate for your fasting days.

Day 1 (Fasting)

Breakfast: Skip breakfast (black coffee, water, tea or sparkling water until noon)

Lunch: Garden salad with grilled chicken (page 206)

Dinner: Chicken and vegetable soup (page 201)

Day 2 (Non-Fasting)

Although this is your "non-fasting" day, I would suggest you stick to the following non-fasting sample meal plan.

Breakfast: Overnight oats with berries (page 192)

Snack: Apple and almond butter (page 236)

Lunch: Four-bean salad (page 204)

Dinner: Grilled halibut with tomato, avocado and mango salsa (page 209)

Day 3 (Fasting)

Breakfast: Skip breakfast (black coffee, water, tea or sparkling water until noon)

Lunch: Roasted cauliflower and spinach salad (page 218)

Dinner: Chicken and vegetable soup (leftover from day one) (page 201)

The Ketogenic Diet (Days 4, 5 and 6)

Reminder: A ketogenic diet is essentially a diet that significantly restricts the amount of carbohydrates you eat each day while increasing fats and consuming moderate protein. Fat consumption should be focused on healthy fats like nuts, seeds, avocado, olive oil, fatty fish and some high-fat dairy (in moderation).

Day 4

Breakfast: Vegetable omelet, 2 slices bacon and 1/4 avocado, sliced (page 195)

Lunch: Greek salad with grilled chicken (page 208)

Snack: 10-15 almonds

Dinner: Salmon and bell pepper stir-fry (page 219)

Day 5

Breakfast: Baked egg and avocado (page 186)

Lunch: BLT lettuce wraps (page 200)

Snack: 1oz hard cheese of your choice

Dinner: Almond-crusted chicken (page 198) with steamed asparagus (page 229)

Day 6

Breakfast: Spinach and bacon frittata (page 193)

Lunch: Avocado, tomato and feta salad (page 199)

Snack: 8 oz full fat sugar-free yogurt

Dinner: Filet mignon and arugula salad (page 203)

The Vegan Diet (Days 7, 8 and 9)

Reminder: A vegan diet avoids all types of foods derived from animals. This naturally includes all animal meats, fish, dairy, and eggs. However, it also includes things like honey, gelatin, and whey. The diet is heavy in vegetables, fresh fruit, nuts, seeds and legumes.

Day 7

Breakfast: Berry protein smoothie with vegan protein powder (page 187)

Lunch: Kale and quinoa salad (page 212)

Snack: Homemade trail mix (page 237)

Dinner: Vegetarian chili (page 224)

Day 8

Breakfast: Overnight oats with berries (page 192)

Lunch: Vegetarian chili (leftover from night before) (page 224)

Snack: Apple and almond butter (page 236)

Dinner: Quinoa and chickpea salad (page 215)

Day 9

Breakfast: Blueberry chia pudding (page 188)

Lunch: Roasted cauliflower and spinach salad
(page 218)

Snack: 10-15 almonds

Dinner: Spaghetti squash with fresh herbs (page 222)

The Mediterranean Diet (Days 10, 11 and 12)

Reminder: The primary foods that make up the Mediterranean diet are fresh vegetables, fish, other seafood, whole grains, healthy oils, unprocessed or un-refined breads, nuts, seeds, legumes, some fruit (in moderation), olive oil and wine. In addition, natural herbs and spices are used to enhance the flavor of the meal. Other proteins like poultry, eggs, and dairy products should be eaten only once a week and in moderate portions. Likewise, red meats should only be eaten on rare occasions, as should sweets and desserts. And unlike other diets, red wine is actually encouraged if you choose.

Day 10

Breakfast: Avocado toast (page 185)

Snack: Apple and almond butter (page 236)

Lunch: Avocado, tomato and feta salad (page 199)

Dinner: Shrimp stir-fry (page 220)

Day 11

Breakfast: Greek yogurt with fresh berries (page 192)

Lunch: Spinach salad with strawberries and walnuts (page 223)

Snack: 10-15 almonds

Dinner: Quinoa stuffed peppers (page 216)

Day 12

Breakfast: Greek frittata (page 191)

Lunch: Quinoa stuffed peppers (left over from night before) (page 216)

Snack: White bean hummus and veggies (page 238)

Dinner: Ginger salmon (page 207) and roasted Brussels sprouts (page 227)

The Low-Calorie Diet (Days 13, 14 and 15)

Reminder: For your Stack, a low-calorie diet is defined as no more than 800 calories a day. (Remember, your stack only lasts three days!) By restricting your calories, instead of only burning food calories from your diet for energy, you start burning calories from stored fats—helping you lose weight fast. During your low-calorie Stack choose foods high in fiber, hydrate well, replace red meat with fish, seafood or lean poultry, consider hot soups and beverages as these also reduce hunger and choose fresh, whole foods rather than processed or refined foods.

Day 13

Breakfast: Vegetable omelet (page 195)

Lunch: Kale, pear and pecan salad (page 214)

Dinner: Chicken and vegetable soup (page 201)

Day 14

Breakfast: Overnight oats with berries (page 192)

Lunch: Chicken and vegetable soup (left over from the night before) (page 201)

Dinner: Spinach salad with strawberries and walnuts (page 223)

Day 15

Breakfast: Green veggie juice (page 190)

Lunch: Quinoa and chickpea salad (page 215)

Dinner: Grilled herb chicken (page 210) with steamed broccoli (page 230)

The Paleo Diet (Days 16, 17, and 18)

Reminder: A Paleo diet, which attempts to mimic the "caveman" diet of our early ancestors, includes foods that hunters and gatherers may come across during their search for food in the wild such as grass-fed meats, fish, seafood, fruits, vegetables, and nuts. Grains, dairy, sugary foods, alcohol and anything processed should be avoided on the Paleo diet.

Day 16

Breakfast: Baked eggs and avocado (page 186)

Lunch: Garden salad with grilled chicken (page 206)

Snack: 10-15 almonds

Dinner: Ginger salmon (page 207) and steamed asparagus (page 229)

Day 17

Breakfast: Veggie scramble with 2 slices bacon (page 196)

Lunch: BLT lettuce wraps (page 200)

Snack: Medium apple

Dinner: Almond-crusted chicken (page 198) and roasted vegetables (page 228)

Day 18

Breakfast: Spinach and bacon frittata (page 193)

Lunch: Kale, pear and pecan salad (page 214)

Snack: Homemade trail mix (page 237)

Dinner: Filet Mignon and arugula salad (page 203)

The Elimination Diet (Days 19, 20 and 21)

There are many ways to do the elimination diet but for the purposes of your Diet Stack, an elimination diet will be defined as a diet that is free of sugar, wheat, dairy, soy, and alcohol.

Day 19

Breakfast: Breakfast tacos (page 189)

Lunch: Kale and quinoa salad (page 212)

Snack: White bean hummus with veggies (page 238)

Dinner: Grilled mahi-mahi with tomato and avocado salsa (page 211)

Day 20

Breakfast: Strawberry coconut chia pudding breakfast bowl (page 194)

Lunch: White chicken stew (page 225)

Snack: Apple and almond butter (page 236)

Dinner: Chicken and wild rice soup (page 202)

Day 21

Breakfast: Green veggie juice (page 190)

Lunch: Chicken and wild rice soup (left over from night before) (page 202)

Snack: ½ cup berries

Dinner: Shrimp stir-fry (page 220)

Extreme Stacking, Extreme Advantages

Choosing the Extreme Stack takes a commitment, but the results are worth the effort. By taking the 21-day Diet Stack Challenge, you will be able to better reach your weight loss goals. But at the same time, each of the Diet Stack diets you choose in your Extreme Stack will promote better overall wellness providing you with more energy and better confidence along the way. This is why many embrace the 21-day Diet Stack Challenge in the pursuit of a healthier life.

CHAPTER 18:

THE CUSTOM STACK

The beauty of the Custom Stack is that you get to choose the specific diets and the duration (number of diets in your Stack) that works best for you. I would suggest starting with one of the pre-determined Stacks as they have been proven to work. But should you be compelled to develop your own Stack or if you have food restrictions that would prevent you from doing one of the pre-developed Stacks, then by all means create your own Custom Stack. You can also use a Custom Stack any time you want to drop a few pounds. For example, I use a Custom 5-Stack after the holidays or following a vacation. Any time I over-indulge and start to see the scale creep up, I can use my Custom Stack to drop the weight quickly and effortlessly.

Follow a few tips when developing your Custom Stack. First, try not to stack diets that are too similar. For example even though keto and Paleo may be in my Stack, I never do them back-to-back. Instead, I Stack diets that are different enough to ensure a feeling of starting fresh which helps peak my motivation and ensure continual weight loss. For example:

Custom Stack example #1: Keto > Vegan > Paleo

Custom Stack example #2: Intermittent Fasting > Mediterranean > Low Cal.

Diets that are too similar don't allow for the "Diet Disruption" which is the foundation of the Diet Stacking program.

When developing your Custom Stack, don't forget to think about what will work best for you. YOU GET TO MAKE THE RULES with the Custom Stack. Don't select a diet that you don't like. And remember, you can put any Diet Stacking approved diet in your Custom Stack as many times as you want. Just make sure that no diet goes more than three days at once. For example, my favorite Custom 10-Stack looks like this:

Dawna's Custom 10-Stack (30 days):

- Intermittent Fasting (Days 1, 2 and 3)
- Keto (Days 4, 5 and 6)
- Vegan (Days 7, 8 and 9)
- Intermittent Fasting (Days 10, 11 and 12)
- Mediterranean (Days 13, 14 and 15)
- Intermittent Fasting (Days 16, 17 and 18)
- Keto (Days 19, 20 and 21)
- Elimination (Days 22, 23 and 24)
- Vegan (Days 25, 26 and 27)
- Intermittent Fasting (Days 28, 20 and 30)

Note: my custom 10-Stack includes intermittent fasting four times, keto and vegan each twice and Mediterranean and elimination each once. Even though other diets may help me lose weight more quickly (take raw or low-calorie for example) the above stack is much easier for me to adhere to and I rarely feel deprived or as if I'm on a diet with this particular stack. It took me a little trial and error and different Custom Stacks to find what worked best for me but once I did, I have a solid plan any time I need to lose weight. Now that I'm near my goal weight, I rarely do a 10-Stack. Instead, I usually do the Simple Stack, also known as the 3-Stack if I overindulge and need to drop a couple pounds.

Should you decide you want to develop your own Custom Stack but have diet restrictions that make some of the diets difficult to follow, remember you can do any of the approved diets more than once during your Stack. For example, if you don't consume meat, you may find it challenging to put the keto or Paleo diets into your stack. In this case, you can double up on the programs that work for your specific wants and needs. For example you may decide to do a 5-Stack that looks like this:

Custom Stack for Non-Meat Eaters:
- Vegan (Days 1, 2 and 3)
- Mediterranean (Days 4, 5 and 6)
- Vegan (Days 7, 8 and 9)
- Intermittent Fasting (Days 10, 11 and 12)
- Raw (Days 13, 14 and 15)

There are unlimited combinations. Do what you know will work best for your specific needs.

As mentioned earlier, if this is your first time Stacking, I encourage you to try one of the pre-developed Stacks, with accompanying meal plans, before developing your own Custom Stack.

You are ready to Stack! Will you do the Simple Stack, Weight Loss Stack, Extreme Stack or Custom Stack? Let's get Stacking!

SECTION IV:
ENSURING SUCCESS

CHAPTER 19:

STACKING RULES

By now, you can appreciate the many advantages that Diet Stacking can provide. For weight loss, each of the Diet Stacks discussed offers you great opportunities to slim down and regain that figure you desire. But at the same time, Diet Stacking offers a way to achieve better health in the process. Not only will you be able to achieve a healthy weight, but you will have more energy and feel better about yourself. And by disrupting the normal dieting process and "Stacking," you will keep a higher level of motivation throughout the program.

As you can appreciate, the Diet Stacking approved diets selected were all carefully researched and studied in an effort to identify ones that offered you the best chance to lose weight while embracing a healthy diet plan. With this in mind, there are a few rules and best practices that should also be followed during your Diet Stacking. In fact, these are excellent dietary habits that should be followed all the time in an effort to be your healthiest. By combining these best practices with the Diet Stack you select, you greatly enhance your chances for success not only now but long-term as well.

It should also be mentioned that these Stacking Rules help you stay on track as you adopt the various Diet Stacks. While each of the Diet Stacking approved diets are uniquely different, the Stacking Rules provide some degree of uniformity among them by encouraging good lifestyle behaviors. As a result, no matter which Diet Stacking approved diet you decide to Stack, these Stacking Rules provide a common thread throughout the program. As a result, you will come to rely of some basic dietary practices that naturally promote a healthy weight and lifestyle. And with this foundation, your chances for success are immense.

DIET STACKING RULES – 10 BEST PRACTICES FOR DIET STACKING SUCCESS

Stacking Rule #1 – Fresh is Best!

Regardless of the Diet Stacking approved diets you have selected, it is important to include as many fresh foods as you can. In fact, fresh, whole foods that are organic in nature offer you the richest sources of nutrients without exposing you to potentially unhealthy substances. When shopping for fruits, vegetables, dairy and other products, choosing fresh, wholesome, organic options should therefore be considered. Exploring farmers' markets and whole-food grocery stores is highly encouraged. Of course, this may not always be available or possible, and the cost of some organic options may not be feasible at times. But whenever you can, select fresh-food offerings. You will not only taste the difference, but you will feel it as well.

Stacking Rule #2 - Avoid the Sugar

As you likely know, sugar is a carbohydrate. Therefore, some Diet Stacking approved diets will naturally limit the amount of carbs you can have as part of their own recommendations. But sugar in general is a carbohydrate that is rapidly absorbed into the blood stream and causes rapid rises in your blood sugar. Why is this bad? Because quick ups and downs in blood sugar levels trigger insulin surges that have been linked to diabetes and weight gain. Plus, these same elevations are known to cause carbohydrate cravings, especially for more sugar. Therefore, for any Diet Stack, avoiding refined sugars as much as possible is important. This not only includes sugary treats but also sugar-sweetened beverages as well. Instead, choose complex carbohydrates and fiber if your Diet Stack allows these foods. Your opportunity for success and for better health will be much higher as a result.

Stacking Rule #3 - Get Rid of Processed Foods

Like refined sugar, processed foods also expose you to unhealthy substances that can undermine your success. Common types of processed foods include those like deli meats, cheese slices, and products containing corn syrup and preservatives. These hidden ingredients, especially high fructose corn syrup, can add empty calories to your diet. And many of these processed foods have unhealthy substances like nitrates and nitrites that can lead to poor health conditions. While you may not be able to avoid processed foods completely, minimizing them in your diet as best as possible is important for both your weight loss and health efforts. All Diet Stacking approved diets embrace this strategy regardless of the food choices allowed.

Stacking Rule #4 – Water is Your Friend

The benefits of staying well hydrated cannot be overstated. For one, drinking water throughout the day helps you feel a bit "fuller," and this can deter some of your hunger while dieting. But also, being well hydrated gives you more energy and allows you to be your best. Why? Simply because our body needs water to function optimally. Your metabolism improves when you're well hydrated, and this helps you lose weight and be more energetic. At the same time, drinking plenty of water helps your body's digestive and urinary systems, which also enhance weight loss and wellness. And of course, water is an excellent replacement for other beverages that might add calories to your daily intake. For all the Diet Stack approved diets, proper hydration is strongly encouraged.

Stacking Rule #5 – How You Prepare Meals Matters

Be smart when preparing your meals. For example, raw foods provide higher levels of nutrition in most cases, which can be an excellent choice at times. When cooking, however, baking, steaming, grilling, broiling and poaching are better choices when compared to basted, fried, or sautéed. And when possible, boost your food's flavor with natural herbs and spices rather than using excessive salt or caloric dressings and sauces. By being smart about how you prepare your meals, you will gain the most out of your Diet Stacking experience.

Stacking Rule #6 – Rules for Restaurants

One of the biggest challenges for anyone trying to stick to a diet involves eating away from home or dining out. Restaurants commonly want to make a big impression on your taste buds, and as a result, many restaurant meals contain a high amount of salt, sugar, and fats. Therefore, developing a smart strategy for dining out is important for any diet including your Diet Stacking approved diets. First of all, don't be afraid of making a special request. Nearly all restaurants are accustomed to making exceptions for food allergies and other special dietary needs. Asking for healthier options is therefore a great strategy when at a restaurant. Other suggestions include asking for sauces and dressings on the side, requesting oil and vinegar dressings instead of creamy ones, and choosing healthier food preparations as discussed in *Stacking Rule #5*. Lastly, splitting a meal with someone, setting aside some to take home, and opting for an appetizer as a meal are additional strategies that may be considered.

Stacking Rule #7 – Coffee, Yes!
Fancy Coffee Drinks, No!

When it comes to coffee, our need for a little morning or mid-afternoon pick-me-up is something many of us enjoy. And in fact, many health studies suggest that coffee in moderation offers some positive health benefits. But as always, the devil is in the details. While coffee itself is perfectly fine to include in your Diet Stacking plans, loading your cup of java with spoonfuls of sugar and cream are not. Avoiding refined sugar (*Stacking Rule #2*) still applies when it comes to your coffee. And avoiding those fancy, delicious-appearing coffee drinks is a must.

Stacking Rule #8 – Cut Back on Alcohol
(Until You Reach Your Goal Weight)

When it comes to alcohol, there are a lot of choices. For example, you may want to have a glass of wine with dinner, or a beer with friends. Or you may want a "hot toddy" on a chilly evening. As a general rule, alcohol should be used in moderation. A glass of red wine with dinner has been shown to promote better heart health, but this certainly does not mean you are required to have one. Likewise, alcohol is highly caloric and offers no real nutritional value. And if the type of alcoholic beverage you choose is loaded with carbs (beer, fruity cocktails), then it might seriously undermine your Diet Stack. Therefore, know which alcoholic drinks are permissible with your Diet Stacking program. And likewise, practice moderation or better yet, skip alcohol during your Stack or at least until you reach your target weight. This will help you stay on track with your weight loss goals.

Stacking Rule #9 – Perform Daily Weigh-Ins

A great way to help maintain your motivation during any diet involves tracking your weight on a daily basis. By seeing your weight start to drop on the scale, you will become increasingly empowered and excited about your Diet Stacking efforts. Remember to weigh yourself at the same time every day (preferably first thing in the morning) and always in the same clothes (or better yet, without clothes). I love using a smart scale as it tracks not only my weight but also my body fat percent and body mass index. Most connect right to your smart phone for easy monitoring over time.

Stacking Rule #10 – Keep a Diet Stacking Journal

As mentioned earlier in the tips for success, journaling is an important activity you should consider. Why? Because journaling helps you better appreciate subtle trends and changes that occur along the way. By appreciating these subtleties, you increase your chances to succeed in losing weight and becoming healthier. For example, journaling can help you identify specific foods that you crave or specific environments where you make poor food choices. Likewise, journaling can help you better understand your emotions and how they influence your food selections. And for Diet Stacking in particular, journaling can help you identify which Diet Stacking approved diets are most effective and enjoyable should you want to build your own Custom Stack in the future.

Get Ready to Stack!

With these 10 stacking rules, and all that you have learned in the previous chapters about the Diet Stacking approved diets, you are now ready to start your Stack. The Diet Stacking rules are meant to help you best achieve the weight loss success you want while also promoting health and wellness. These are important regardless of the Diet Stack you select. It is also important to stick to the guidelines provided for each of the individual Diet Stacking approved diets in your program. Remember, each diet in your Stack should last just three days. And the charts of foods to include and avoid as well as the detailed meal plans should guide your meal choices during that time. By taking this approach, you will give yourself the best opportunity to realize your weight loss goals. Here's to you and to your Diet Stacking success!

CHAPTER 20:
POST STACK

When you lose weight, there is often fear of regaining it. Don't worry! You got this! Not only will it be easier to lost weight with Stacking, but you can also utilize your new-found Stacking knowledge to drop a few unwanted pounds whenever needed.

Once your Stack is done, there are several things you can do to ensure the weight you lost during your Stack stays off. There are also several ways to continue to use Diet Stacking to ward off unwanted weight gain or to lose weight following a vacation, the holiday season, or anything that may cause you to add a few extra-unwanted pounds.

First, continue to adhere to the 10 same rules that were outlined in Chapter 19 as you did while on your stack. Second, use shorter or customized stacks any time you need to lose a few pounds. Third, cook once and eat twice (or even three times). That is, prepare your meals in advance whenever you can and make enough for two to three days. Planning your meals for the week and more importantly preparing your meals ahead of time will help you stay on track and help you avoid picking up the first unhealthy thing you see when hunger or cravings hit.

Lastly, be kind to yourself. Allow yourself to indulge on occasion and in moderation. Listen to your body and give it healthy, fresh and unprocessed foods 90% of the time!

You can do it!

Want to stack with me? Join the Diet Stacking Online Challenge. Go to DawnaStone.com/DietStacking to find out more and sign up.

APPENDIX I:
DIET STACKING RECIPES

TABLE OF CONTENTS

BREAKFAST RECIPES

AVOCADO TOAST

Works with: Intermittent Fasting | Vegan | Mediterranean

Ingredients:

1 hardboiled egg, chopped into small pieces (optional)*
½ ripe avocado, pitted, peeled and cubed
Juice of ½ lemon
¼ teaspoon sea salt
1/8 teaspoon black pepper
2 slices sourdough bread
2 radishes, thinly sliced

Directions:

Hard boil the egg by filling a pot halfway with water and insert egg (make sure egg is covered by at least one inch). Bring water to a boil over high heat. Once the water boils, remove the pan from the heat, cover and let the egg sit for 8-10 minutes. Remove the egg from the pot and cool in ice water for several minutes. Peel the egg and set aside.

In a small bowl, combine the avocado, lemon juice, sea salt and pepper. Smash together.

Spread avocado mixture onto sourdough toast. Chop hardboiled egg and spread over avocado. Top with radish slices and serve.

MAKES 2 SERVINGS

*Eliminate egg for vegan option

BAKED EGG AND AVOCADO

Works with: Intermittent Fasting | Ketogenic | Low-Carb | Paleo |
Elimination | Anti-Inflammatory | Mediterranean | Low-Calorie

Ingredients:

1 ripe avocado, halved and pitted
2 eggs
½ teaspoon sea salt
¼ teaspoon black pepper

Directions:

Preheat over to 425°F.

To allow room for the egg, scoop out an additional tablespoon or two from the center of each avocado half.

Place avocado on a small baking dish lined with parchment paper and crack an egg into each half.

Bake for 15-20 minutes or until egg whites have set and yolk is still runny. Remove from oven and add salt and pepper.

MAKES 2 SERVINGS

BERRY PROTEIN SMOOTHIE

Works with: Intermittent Fasting | Elimination | Anti-Inflammatory | Vegan | Low-Calorie

Ingredients:

1 scoop high quality pea protein powder
1 cup unsweetened plain almond milk
½ cup frozen berries (strawberries, blackberries and/or blueberries)
2 ice cubes

Directions:

In a blender, combine pea protein powder, almond milk, berries and ice.

MAKES 1 SERVING

BLUEBERRY CHIA PUDDING

Works with: Intermittent Fasting | Vegan | Mediterranean

Ingredients:

1 cup unsweetened plain almond milk
1 cup plain Greek yogurt (or non-dairy yogurt*)
¼ cup chia seeds
2 tablespoons honey (or agave nectar*)
1 cup fresh blueberries

Directions:

In a medium bowl combine almond milk, yogurt, chia seeds and honey. Whisk until mixed well.

Let stand at room temperature for 20-30 minutes, cover and refrigerate overnight.

When ready to eat, divide chia mixture into two glass jars or small bowls, top with fresh blueberries and serve.

MAKES 2 SERVINGS

Use non-dairy yogurt and agave nectar in this recipe for the vegan diet

BREAKFAST TACOS

Works with: Intermittent Fasting | Elimination

Ingredients:

4 large eggs
4 corn tortillas
Olive oil spray
1 tablespoon diced onion
¼ cup tomato, diced
¼ jalapeño, diced
1 cup baby spinach, stems removed
¼ cup queso fresco, crumbled*
½ teaspoon salt
¼ teaspoon black pepper
Hot sauce, to taste (optional)

Directions:

In a mixing bowl, whisk the eggs.

Lightly char each tortilla by placing them in a pan over medium high heat. Flip the tortilla often so it doesn't burn. Remove when tortilla begins to show light brown spots. Reserve tortillas.

Coat a medium skillet with olive oil spray. Add onion and cook for 1 to 2 minutes or until translucent. Add the tomato, jalapeño and spinach and cook for 1 minute or until spinach is wilted. Pour in the eggs and cook for 3 to 4 minutes or until desired doneness. Remove from heat.

Top the four tortillas with egg mixture. Add queso, salt, pepper and hot sauce (optional).

MAKES 4 TACOS

Remove cheese for the elimination diet

GREEN VEGGIE JUICE

Works with: Intermittent Fasting | Low-carb | Raw | Elimination |
Anti-Inflammatory | Vegan | Mediterranean | Low-Calorie

Ingredients:

1 cup baby spinach, stems removed
1 green apple, core removed
1 rib celery
½ cucumber
½ lemon
1-inch piece fresh ginger

Directions:

In a juicer, juice the spinach, apple, celery, cucumber, lemon and
ginger. Pour over ice and enjoy.

MAKES 1 SERVING

GREEK FRITTATA

*Works with: Ketogenic | Low-Carb | Paleo | Mediterranean |
Low-Calorie*

Ingredients:

8 large eggs
2 cups fresh baby spinach leaves, stems removed
2 tomatoes, chopped
½ cup mushrooms, sliced
½ green bell pepper, diced
½ cup red onion, finely chopped
¼ cup feta, crumbled (optional*)
1 tablespoon fresh basil, chopped
¼ teaspoon sea salt
¼ teaspoon ground black pepper
1 tablespoon extra-virgin olive oil

Directions:

Preheat the oven to 400°F.

In a mixing bowl, whisk the eggs. Fold in the spinach, tomatoes, mushrooms, bell pepper, onion and feta. Stir in the basil, salt, and pepper.

Coat a large ovenproof, skillet with the olive oil and heat over medium heat.

Pour the egg mixture into the skillet and cook until the eggs start to set (approximately 1 minute).

Transfer the skillet to the oven and bake for 5 to 6 minutes, or until the top is lightly browned.

Remove the frittata from the oven and let it stand for 5 minutes before cutting and serving.

MAKES 4 SERVINGS

Leave out feta for paleo diet

GREEK YOGURT WITH FRESH BERRIES

Works with: Intermittent Fasting | Vegan | Mediterranean | Low-Calorie

Ingredients:

1 cup Greek yogurt (or non-dairy yogurt*)
3 strawberries, sliced

Directions:

In a bowl, top Greek yogurt with berries and enjoy!

MAKES 1 SERVING

*Use non-dairy yogurt for vegan diet

OVERNIGHT OATS WITH BERRIES

Works with: Intermittent Fasting | Elimination | Anti-Inflammatory | Vegan | Mediterranean | Low-Calorie

Ingredients:

½ cup gluten-free oats
1 cup unsweetened almond milk
2 strawberries, sliced
½ tablespoon sliced almonds

Directions:

In a jar, combine oats and almond milk. Cover and refrigerate overnight. In the morning, top with strawberries and almonds.

MAKES 1 SERVING

SPINACH AND BACON FRITTATA

Works with: Ketogenic | Low-Carb | Paleo | Mediterranean

Ingredients:

8 large eggs
2 cups fresh baby spinach leaves, stems removed
2 tomatoes, chopped
½ cup red onion, finely chopped
4 slices thick cut bacon, pre-cooked and crumbled
1 teaspoon dried thyme
¼ teaspoon sea salt
¼ teaspoon ground black pepper
1 tablespoon extra-virgin olive oil

Directions:

Preheat the oven to 400°F. In a mixing bowl, whisk the eggs. Fold in the spinach, tomatoes, onion and bacon. Stir in the thyme, salt, and pepper.

Coat a large ovenproof, skillet with the olive oil and heat over medium heat. Pour the egg mixture into the skillet and cook until the eggs start to set (approximately 1 minute).

Transfer the skillet to the oven and bake for 5 to 6 minutes, or until the top is lightly browned. Remove the frittata from the oven and let it stand for 5 minutes before cutting and serving.

MAKES 4 SERVINGS

STRAWBERRY COCONUT CHIA PUDDING BREAKFAST BOWL

Works with: Intermittent Fasting | Elimination | Vegan | Mediterranean

Ingredients:

Pudding:

1 tablespoon chia seeds
1 cup almond milk
1 cup plain full fat Greek yogurt (or non-dairy option*)
1 tablespoon honey (or maple syrup*)

Topping:

4 strawberries, sliced
1 tablespoon sliced almonds
1 tablespoon unsweetened coconut flakes
1 teaspoon flax seeds

Directions:

Mix pudding ingredients and refrigerate for at least 30-45 minutes (or overnight). Top with strawberries, almonds, coconut and flax and enjoy!

MAKES 1 SERVING

*Use a non-dairy substitute for the vegan diet

VEGETABLE OMELET

Works with: Intermittent Fasting | Ketogenic | Low-carb | Paleo |
Elimination | Mediterranean | Low-Calorie

Ingredients:

2 large eggs
2 teaspoon extra-virgin olive oil
1 tablespoon sweet onion, thinly chopped
1 small tomato, chopped
3 small button mushrooms, sliced
½ cup fresh baby spinach leaves, stems removed
¼ teaspoon sea salt
1/8 teaspoon black pepper

Directions:

In a small bowl, whisk the eggs and set aside.

Coat a small nonstick skillet with 1 teaspoon olive oil and heat over medium heat.

Cook the onion for 1 minute or until translucent. Toss in the tomato and mushrooms and cook for an additional 4 to 5 minutes, or until tender. Transfer vegetables to a bowl.

Clean the skillet and coat with the remaining teaspoon of olive oil. Set over medium-high

heat. Add the reserved eggs and cook for 2 minutes (do not stir).

As the center sets, transfer the cooked vegetables to one side of the omelet. Top with the spinach. Season with salt and pepper. Gently fold 1 side of the omelet over the other.

Cook for 1 minute to let set. Remove from skillet and serve.

MAKES 1 SERVING

VEGGIE SCRAMBLE

Works with: Intermittent Fasting | Ketogenic | Low-Carb | Paleo |
Elimination | Mediterranean | Low-Calorie

Ingredients:

2 large eggs
¼ teaspoon salt
1/8 teaspoon black pepper
1 teaspoon extra-virgin olive oil
¼ cup onions, diced
½ cup baby spinach, stems removed
½ cup tomatoes, chopped
¼ cup orange or green bell pepper

Directions:

Whisk the eggs in a bowl. Add salt and pepper and set aside.

Coat a small nonstick skillet with the olive oil and place over medium heat. Cook the onions 1 to 2 minutes or until translucent. Add the spinach, tomatoes and bell pepper and cook for 2 minutes, or until the spinach is wilted. Pour the reserved eggs over the vegetables.

Cook the eggs and vegetables for 1 to 3 minutes, stirring gently, until desired doneness.

MAKES 1 SERVING

LUNCH AND DINNER RECIPES

ALMOND CRUSTED CHICKEN

Works with: Intermittent Fasting | Ketogenic | Low-Carb | Paleo | Elimination | Mediterranean

Ingredients:

¾ cup almond meal
¼ teaspoon paprika
½ teaspoon onion powder
½ teaspoon oregano
2 teaspoon sea salt
½ teaspoon garlic powder
2 eggs
4 boneless, skinless chicken breasts
2 tablespoon extra virgin olive oil

Directions:

In a large bowl, combine the almond meal, paprika, onion powder, oregano, salt and garlic powder and set aside.

In a medium bowl, whisk the eggs and set aside.

Pound the chicken to an even thickness (about ½ inch) by placing the breasts between 2 plastic bags or sheets of plastic wrap and hitting the thick part of the chicken with a flat meat pounder or rolling pin.

Dip the chicken breasts into the egg mixture. After dipping chicken into the egg, dip into the dry mixture so that it is evenly covered.

In a deep skillet, heat the oil on medium-high heat. Add the chicken to the skillet and cook for 6 to 8 minutes on each side or until cooked through. Time will depend on the thickness of the chicken.

MAKES 4 SERVINGS

AVOCADO, TOMATO AND FETA SALAD

Works with: Intermittent Fasting | Ketogenic | Low-Carb | Mediterranean

Ingredients:

2 tomatoes, seeded and diced
1 avocado, peeled pitted and cubed
½ cup red onion, finely chopped
¼ cup fresh cilantro, chopped
2 tablespoons freshly squeezed lemon juice
¼ teaspoon salt to taste
¼ cup feta cheese, crumbled
1 tablespoon extra virgin olive oil

Directions:

In medium bowl, combine all ingredients, and let stand for 15 to 20 minutes.

MAKES 2 SERVINGS

BLT LETTUCE WRAPS

Works with: Intermittent Fasting | Ketogenic | Low-Carb | Paleo | Mediterranean

Ingredients:

2 romaine lettuce leaf or other leafy green like butter lettuce
2 slices bacon
2 slices tomato

Directions:

In a skillet (or microwave) cook bacon to desired doneness and set aside. For an open faced BLT, top each lettuce leaf with one slice tomato and one slice of bacon.

MAKES 1 SERVING

CHICKEN AND VEGETABLE SOUP

Works with: Intermittent Fasting | Ketogenic | Low-Carb | Paleo | Elimination | Anti-Inflammatory | Mediterranean | Low-Calorie

Ingredients:

1 tablespoon extra virgin olive oil
½ onion diced
1 clove garlic
2 carrots, sliced
4 cups chicken broth
1 can diced tomatoes
4 celery stalks, sliced
1 zucchini, spiralized or chopped
2 cups spinach, stems removed
1 rotisserie chicken breast, shredded (already cooked)

Directions:

Heat the oil in a Dutch oven medium-high heat. Add the onion and garlic, stirring frequently for 3-4 minutes or until the onion is translucent. Add the carrots and stir for 1 minute. Add the broth, canned tomatoes, celery and zucchini. Bring to a boil, reduce heat and simmer for 12-15 minutes or until vegetables are tender. Add the spinach and shredded chicken and simmer for an additional 10 minutes.

MAKES 2 SERVINGS

CHICKEN AND WILD RICE SOUP

Works with: Intermittent Fasting | Elimination | Anti-Inflammatory | Mediterranean | Low-Calorie

Ingredients:

1 cup uncooked wild rice
2 tablespoon extra virgin olive oil
½ onion, chopped
1 clove garlic, minced
6 cups organic, low sodium chicken broth
2 carrots, chopped
2 celery stalks, chopped
2 medium tomatoes, seeded and chopped
2 sprigs thyme
salt, to taste
pepper, to taste
1 rotisserie chicken, skin and bones removed (already cooked)
2 cups spinach, stems removed
Italian parsley for garnish (optional)

Directions:

Cook rice according to package directions and set aside.

In a large Dutch oven, heat the olive oil over medium-high heat. Add onion and garlic and sauté for 3 minutes or until onions begin to turn translucent. Add broth, carrots, celery, tomatoes, and thyme and bring to a boil. Cover, reduce heat and simmer for 5 minutes. Add salt, pepper, reserved rice, chicken, and spinach and simmer for 8 to 10 minutes or until chicken is warmed through.

Remove thyme sprigs. Top with parsley and serve.

MAKES 6 SERVINGS

FILET MIGNON AND ARUGULA SALAD

Works with: Intermittent Fasting | Ketogenic | Low-Carb | Paleo | Mediterranean

Ingredients:

½ pound filet mignon (two 4 oz steaks)
¼ teaspoon coarse salt
¼ ground black pepper
2 cups pre-washed arugula
2 tablespoons white balsamic vinaigrette (see recipe in dressing section)

Directions:

Preheat grill to medium-high heat. Season filet with salt and pepper and grill 4-5 minutes on each side or until desired temperature. Let cool slightly (5-10 minutes). Slice steak thinly, and place over arugula. Drizzle with white balsamic vinaigrette.

MAKES 2 SERVINGS

FOUR-BEAN SALAD

*Works with: Intermittent Fasting | Elimination | Anti-
Inflammatory | Vegan | Mediterranean*

Ingredients:

Salad:

2 cups yellow wax beans, cut in half and trimmed
2 cups green beans, cut in half and trimmed
4 radishes, washed and sliced thin
1 cup garbanzo beans
1 cup northern beans (or any white bean)
¼ cup roughly chopped fresh dill

Dressing:

½ cup extra virgin olive oil
¼ cup white balsamic vinegar
½ teaspoon sea salt
¼ teaspoon ground black pepper

Directions:

For the dressing, whisk together the vinegar, oil, salt and pepper
in a medium bowl and set aside (or use any of the dressings in this
appendix).

In a large pot with a tight-fitting lid, place a steamer tray in the pot
and add enough cold water to cover the bottom of the pot by about
1-2 inches. Cover the pot and bring the water to a boil. Add the
yellow and green beans and lower the heat to a simmer. Steam the
vegetables to a tender-crisp and take care not to overcook.

continued...

While the vegetables are steaming prepare an ice bath (large bowl of water with ice cubes). When the vegetables are done, drain with a strainer and immediately place in the ice bath. Once cooled, remove from ice bath and set aside.

In a large bowl combine yellow beans, green beans, radishes, garbanzo beans, northern beans, and dill. Gently mix, top with dressing and serve.

MAKES 4 SERVINGS

GARDEN SALAD WITH GRILLED CHICKEN

Works with: Intermittent Fasting | Ketogenic | Low-carb | Paleo |
Elimination | Mediterranean | Low-calorie

Ingredients:

1 boneless, skinless chicken breast (organic or hormone-free
  preferred)
Pinch of salt
Pinch of ground black pepper
2 cups romaine lettuce, torn into bite-size pieces
1 small tomato, sliced
4 thin slices, red onion
¼ cucumber, sliced
2 tablespoons white balsamic vinaigrette (see recipe in dressing
  section)

Directions:

Prepare grill, or preheat broiler. Season chicken with salt and pepper.
Grill or broil chicken for 15-20 minutes, turning once or until no
trace of pink remains. Cut chicken into strips.

Wash and place salad and remaining ingredients in bowl and toss
with dressing. Top with chicken.

MAKES 1 SERVING

GINGER SALMON

Works with: Intermittent Fasting | Ketogenic | Low-Carb | Paleo | Elimination | Anti-Inflammatory | Mediterranean | Low-Calorie

Ingredients:

1 teaspoon fresh ginger, minced
2 tablespoons reduced-sodium soy sauce or tamari (gluten-free/ wheat-free)*
2 (4-oz) salmon fillets, skin removed
Extra virgin olive oil spray
1 teaspoon toasted sesame seeds

Directions:

Combine ginger and soy sauce in large sealable plastic bag. Add fish, and shake gently to coat. Place in refrigerator. Preheat broiler. Place fish on broiler pan coated with cooking spray. Broil 13-15 minutes, or until fish flakes easily with fork.

Sprinkle with sesame seeds.

MAKES 2 SERVINGS

Use gluten-free options for keto, paleo, elimination and anti-inflammatory diets

GREEK SALAD WITH GRILLED CHICKEN

Works with: Intermittent Fasting | Ketogenic | Low-Carb | Vegan | Mediterranean

Ingredients:

2 boneless, skinless chicken breasts
Salt, to taste
Pepper, to taste
4 cups romaine lettuce, torn into bite-size pieces
1 tomato, sliced
8-10 Kalamata olives
½ cucumber, seeded and chopped
¼ cup red onion, finely chopped
¼ cup feta cheese, crumbled (optional)*
2 tablespoons Greek dressing (see recipe in dressing section)

Directions:

Prepare grill or preheat broiler. Season chicken with salt and pepper. Grill or broil chicken for 15-20 minutes, turning once, or until no trace of pink remains. Cut chicken into strips.

Combine lettuce, tomato, olives, cucumber, and red onion in large bowl. Sprinkle with feta and toss with Greek dressing. Top with chicken and serve.

MAKES 2 SERVINGS

Eliminate feta for vegan diet

GRILLED HALIBUT WITH TOMATO, AVOCADO AND MANGO SALSA

Works with: Intermittent Fasting | Ketogenic | Low-Carb | Paleo | Elimination | Anti-Inflammatory | Mediterranean | Low-Calorie

Ingredients:

Salsa

1 tomato, seeded and diced
½ cup ripe mango, peeled and diced (optional*)
4 cups red onion, finely chopped
¼ cup fresh cilantro, chopped
2 tablespoons freshly squeezed lime juice
¼ teaspoon salt
Ground black pepper to taste

Fish

2 (6 oz) halibut filets
½ tablespoon extra virgin olive oil
Salt
Pepper
1 lime

Directions:

In medium bowl, combine first 7 tomato-mango salsa ingredients, and let stand for 15 to 20 minutes.

Preheat grill or broiler, lightly brush halibut with olive oil, and season with salt and pepper. Place fish on grill or in broiler. Cook 5 to 7 minutes per side (make sure fish is opaque at its center).

Top fish with salsa and serve.

MAKES 4 SERVINGS

Eliminate mango for keto diet

GRILLED HERB CHICKEN

Works with: Intermittent Fasting | Ketogenic | Low-Carb | Paleo | Elimination | Anti-Inflammatory | Mediterranean | Low-Calorie

Ingredients:

4 boneless, skinless chicken breasts (organic or hormone-free preferred)
1 tablespoon extra virgin olive oil
1 teaspoon dried oregano
1 teaspoon thyme
1 teaspoon rosemary
½ teaspoon salt
¼ teaspoon garlic, minced

Directions:

Preheat grill on medium heat. Lightly oil grates so chicken doesn't stick. Rinse chicken, and place in large re-sealable plastic bag with olive oil. Seal, and shake. Open bag, and add ingredients. Shake bag to coat chicken. Cook chicken approximately 7-10 minutes on each side, or until thoroughly cooked.

Note: If you don't have access to a grill, place chicken in a grill pan.

MAKES 4 SERVINGS

GRILLED MAHI-MAHI WITH TOMATO AND AVOCADO SALSA

Works with: Intermittent Fasting | Ketogenic | Low-Carb | Paleo | Raw | Elimination | Anti-Inflammatory | Mediterranean | Low-Calorie

Ingredients:

Salsa

½ tomato, pitted and chopped
½ avocado, peeled, pitted and chopped
1 tablespoon fresh lemon juice (approximately half a lemon)
¼ teaspoon sea salt

Fish

2 6oz mahi-mahi fillets
½ tablespoon olive oil
½ teaspoon sea salt
¼ teaspoon ground black pepper

Directions:

In a small bowl combine the tomato, avocado and lemon juice. Sprinkle with sea salt and set aside.

Brush the fish with olive oil (any remaining oil can be placed in the grill pan) and season with salt and pepper. Heat a grill pan on medium-high and grill for approximately 5 to 7 minutes on each side, or until the fish flakes easily. (the thickness of the fish will determine the exact cooking time needed)

Serve with fresh vegetables or over mixed greens.

MAKES 2 SERVINGS

KALE AND QUINOA SALAD

Works with: Intermittent Fasting | Elimination | Anti-Inflammatory | Vegan | Mediterranean

Ingredients:

Salad:

¾ cup red quinoa

1 ½ cup water

1 teaspoon salt

½ bunch kale, washed, stems removed and chopped

1 carrot, chopped

1 tomato, chopped

½ cucumber, chopped

½ yellow pepper, chopped

¼ red onion, chopped

1 tablespoon sliced almonds

Dressing (or use any of the dressing recipes in this appendix)

½ cup extra virgin olive oil

1 tablespoon balsamic vinegar

1 teaspoon salt

¼ teaspoon black pepper

1 teaspoon Dijon mustard

Directions:

Combine quinoa, water and salt in a saucepan. Bring to a boil, reduce heat and simmer on low until water is absorbed (approximately 15 minutes). Remove from heat and keep covered.

To make the dressing, whisk together olive oil, balsamic vinegar, salt, pepper and Dijon mustard in a small bowl and set aside.

continued...

In a large bowl combine kale, carrots, tomato, cucumber, pepper and onion. Fold in the quinoa and gently stir.

Split between two bowls, sprinkle with sliced almonds and drizzle with dressing.

MAKES 2 SERVINGS

KALE, PEAR AND PECAN SALAD

Works with: Intermittent Fasting | Low-carb | Raw | Elimination | Anti-Inflammatory Vegan | Mediterranean

Ingredients:

4 cups kale, stems removed
½ fennel bulb, thinly sliced (optional)
½ pear, sliced
¼ cup pecans, roughly chopped
¼ cup red onion, thinly sliced
2 tablespoons white balsamic vinaigrette (see recipe in dressing
    section)

Directions:

In bowl, combine kale, fennel, pear, pecans and red onion. Toss with white balsamic vinaigrette.

MAKES 2 SERVINGS

QUINOA AND CHICKPEA SALAD

Works with: Intermittent Fasting | Elimination | Anti-Inflammatory | Vegan | Mediterranean | Low-Calorie

Ingredients:

Salad:

½ cup quinoa

½ cup chickpeas

½ cup red kidney beans

1 carrot, sliced thin

2 celery stalks, sliced thin

1 teaspoon sea salt

Dressing:

2 tablespoon extra virgin olive oil

1 tablespoon balsamic vinegar

½ teaspoon sea salt

¼ teaspoon black pepper

½ teaspoon dried oregano

Directions:

Cook quinoa according to package directions. Cover and refrigerate until chilled.

Add the chickpeas, beans, carrots, celery, and sea salt to the quinoa and toss to mix.

In a small bowl, whisk together the olive oil, balsamic vinegar, sea salt, black pepper, and oregano. Pour the dressing over the quinoa mixture and toss well to combine. The salad can be stored in the refrigerator for 2 to 3 days. You can also choose any of the salad dressing recipes in this appendix.

MAKES 2 SERVINGS

QUINOA STUFFED PEPPERS

Works with: Intermittent Fasting | Elimination | Anti-Inflammatory | Vegan | Mediterranean

Ingredients:

1 ½ cups quinoa
3 cups vegetable broth
1 tablespoon extra virgin olive oil, plus more for preparing baking pan
½ small yellow onion, diced
1 large carrot, diced
2 cloves garlic, minced
1 teaspoon cumin
1 teaspoon dried oregano
1 teaspoon sea salt
½ teaspoon black pepper
⅓ cup sliced almonds
4 red or yellow bell peppers, cored, seeded and halved (reserve top of pepper)

Directions:

Preheat the oven to 400°F.

In a saucepan over medium-high heat, combine the quinoa and broth and bring to a boil. Reduce the heat to low, cover, and cook for about 15 minutes, or until the broth is absorbed. Fluff with a fork and set aside.

In a Dutch oven over medium-high heat, heat the oil. Add the onion and cook, stirring frequently, for 4 to 5 minutes, or until translucent. Add the carrots, and garlic, and cook stirring frequently for 1 minute. Add the reserved quinoa, cumin, oregano, salt, pepper, and almonds and cook for 1 to 2 minutes more. Set aside to let filling cool until slightly warm.

continued...

Oil a 9x12 baking pan. Divide the quinoa mixture evenly among the bell peppers. Place the reserved top on each pepper and arrange them upright in the pan. Cover the peppers with foil and bake for approximately 30-40 minutes or until peppers are tender and filling is hot throughout. Transfer to plates and serve.

MAKES 4 SERVINGS

ROASTED CAULIFLOWER AND SPINACH SALAD

Works with: Intermittent Fasting | Low-Carb | Elimination | Anti-Inflammatory | Vegan | Mediterranean

Ingredients:

1 head cauliflower, cut into bite-size pieces
2 tablespoons extra virgin olive oil
2 teaspoon sea salt
2 cups spinach, stems removed
1 carrot, chopped
2 dates, pitted and chopped
1 tablespoon pine nuts

Dressing:

¼ cup olive oil
1 tablespoon balsamic vinegar
½ teaspoon sea salt
¼ teaspoon

Directions:

Preheat over to 400 degrees. Place cauliflower on a baking tray and drizzle with extra virgin olive oil. Add salt.

Roast for 12-15 minutes or until cauliflower is tender.

In a small bowl, whisk together olive oil, vinegar, salt and pepper and set aside.

In a medium to large bowl, combine spinach, carrots, dates and pine nuts. Top with roasted cauliflower and toss with dressing.

MAKES 2 SERVINGS

SALMON AND BELL PEPPER STIR FRY

Works with: Intermittent Fasting | Ketogenic | Low-Carb | Paleo | Raw | Elimination | Anti-Inflammatory | Vegan | Mediterranean

Ingredients:

Sauce

1 teaspoon honey (optional)*
2 tablespoons tamari
2 tablespoons vegetable stock

Stir-Fry

2 tablespoons sesame oil
1 pound salmon fillet
1 clove garlic, minced
3 bell peppers (yellow, orange and red), seeded and sliced
2 teaspoon minced ginger
1 teaspoon sesame seeds

Directions:

To make the sauce: In a small bowl, combine honey, tamari, and vegetable stock and mix well. Set aside.

To make the stir-fry: In a large skillet over medium-high heat, heat the oil and swirl the pan to coat. Cook salmon for 2 minutes on each side (salmon will not be completely done). Remove salmon and set aside. Add garlic to the pan stirring consistently for 1 to 2 minutes. Add bell peppers and pour on reserved sauce mixture and cook, stirring constantly, for 3 to 4 minutes. Add ginger and reserved salmon and cook for an additional 2 to 3 minutes or until salmon is done and bell peppers are tender. Sprinkle with sesame seeds and serve.

MAKES 4 SERVINGS

*Eliminate honey for keto, paleo and vegan diets

SHRIMP STIR-FRY

Works with: Intermittent Fasting | Elimination | Mediterranean | Low–Calorie

Ingredients:

Sauce

2 tablespoons tamari
2 tablespoons vegetable stock

Stir-Fry

¾ cup quinoa, rinsed and drained (optional*)
1.5 cups water (optional*)
2 tablespoons sesame oil
1 pound medium shrimp, peeled and deveined
2 green onions, chopped
1 clove garlic, minced
½ head cabbage, chopped or shredded
2/3 cup shredded carrots
2 cups snow peas
2 teaspoon minced ginger

Directions:

To make the sauce: In a small bowl, combine the tamari, and vegetable stock and mix well. Set aside.

To make the quinoa (optional): In a saucepan over medium-high heat, combine the quinoa and water and bring to a boil. Reduce the heat to low, cover, and cook for 15 minutes, or until the water is absorbed. Set aside, covered, to steam for 5 minutes. Fluff the quinoa with a fork and transfer to a bowl. Set aside.

To make the stir-fry: In a large skillet over medium-high heat, heat the oil and swirl the pan to coat. Cook shrimp for 1 minute on each side (shrimp will not be completely done). Remove shrimp and set aside. Add onions and garlic to the pan stirring consistently for 1 to 2 minutes. Add cabbage, carrots, and snow peas, and pour on reserved sauce mixture and cook, stirring constantly, for 2 to 3 minutes. Add ginger and shrimp and cook for an additional 2 to 3 minutes or until shrimp is done.

Fluff the reserved quinoa with a fork and divide it among 4 plates. Spoon the stir-fry mixture over the quinoa and serve.

MAKES 4 SERVINGS

Remove if eliminating quinoa from the recipe

SPAGHETTI SQUASH WITH FRESH HERBS

Works with: Intermittent Fasting | Elimination | Anti-Inflammatory | Vegan | Mediterranean

Ingredients:

1 medium spaghetti squash
1 tablespoon extra virgin olive oil
1 clove garlic, minced
1 medium tomato, chopped
1 tablespoon fresh basil, minced
¼ cup pine nuts
¼ cup grated Parmesan cheese (optional*)
sea salt
pepper

Directions:

Pre-heat the oven to 375°F.

Pierce the squash in several places with a fork. Microwave whole squash on high for 10 minutes. Place whole squash on glass baking sheet and roast for 1 hour or until tender.

Let cool for 5 to 10 minutes, cut in half lengthwise and scrape the insides with a fork to remove the long strands of flesh. Transfer to a bowl.

In a skillet, heat 1 tablespoon olive oil over medium heat. Add garlic and sauté for 1 minute. Add tomatoes and sauté for 1 minute. Turn off heat and add spaghetti squash, basil, oregano and salt. Gently combine ingredients.

Divide between two bowls and top with pine nuts and cheese and salt and pepper to taste.

MAKES 2 SERVINGS

*Remove cheese for elimination, anti-inflammatory and vegan diets**

SPINACH SALAD WITH STRAWBERRIES AND WALNUTS

Works with: Intermittent Fasting | Raw | Elimination | Anti-Inflammatory | Vegan | Mediterranean | Low-Calorie

<u>Ingredients:</u>

4 cups spinach, stems removed
4 strawberries sliced
¼ cup walnuts roughly chopped
¼ cup red onion, thinly sliced
2 tablespoons walnut vinaigrette (see recipe in dressing section)

<u>Directions:</u>

In bowl, combine spinach, strawberries, walnuts and red onion. Toss with walnut vinaigrette.

MAKES 2 SERVINGS

VEGETARIAN CHILI

*Works with: Elimination | Anti-Inflammatory | Vegan |
Mediterranean*

Ingredients

1 tablespoon extra-virgin olive oil
½ red onion, finely chopped
1 clove garlic, minced
2 stalks celery, chopped
1 teaspoon chili powder
1 teaspoon cumin
1 teaspoon ground coriander
½ teaspoon sea salt
1 cup crushed tomatoes
1 cup water
1 cup garbanzo beans, cooked and drained
1 cup black beans, cooked and drained
1 cup kidney beans, cooked and drained
2 tablespoon hot sauce
¼ cup chopped cilantro

Directions:

In a large saucepan over medium heat, heat the oil. Cook the onion
until softened (approximately 3-4 minutes). Add the garlic and cook
for an additional 3 minutes. Add the celery, chili powder, cumin,
coriander and sea salt. Stir until combined. Add the tomatoes, water
and beans and bring to a boil. Reduce heat, cover and simmer for
20 minutes.

Add hot sauce to taste and garnish with cilantro.

MAKES 4 SERVINGS

WHITE CHICKEN STEW

Works with: Intermittent Fasting | Elimination | Mediterranean | Low-Calorie

Ingredients:

2 tablespoons extra virgin olive oil
1 clove garlic, minced
1 yellow onion, chopped
2 ribs celery, chopped
1 large (or 3 small) carrots, peeled and chopped
sea salt
ground black pepper
1 yellow pepper, chopped
1 jalapeño, diced (optional)
½ Anaheim pepper, diced
1 can diced green chilies
6 cups chicken broth
1 cans northern beans
1 cup chopped kale
1 rotisserie chicken, boned, skinned and coarsely chopped

Directions:

In a Dutch oven, heat the oil over medium-high heat. Add the garlic, onion, celery, and carrots. Sauté for approximately 5 minutes or until the onion is translucent. Add salt and pepper.

Add the yellow pepper, jalapeño, Anaheim pepper, and green chilies and cook an additional 3-5 minutes. Add the broth, beans and kale. Bring to a boil, reduce the heat, and simmer for 25 minutes, or until the vegetables are tender. Add chicken and simmer an additional 5 to 10 minutes or until chicken is warmed through.

MAKES 4 SERVINGS

SIDES

ROASTED BRUSSELS SPROUTS

Works with: Intermittent Fasting | Ketogenic | Low-Carb | Paleo | Elimination | Anti-Inflammatory | Vegan | Mediterranean | Low-Calorie

Ingredients:

1 cup Brussels sprouts, halved
Extra virgin olive oil
Salt
Pepper

Directions:

Pre-heat oven to 450 degrees. Place Brussels sprouts on a baking tray and drizzle with extra virgin olive oil. Add salt and pepper.

Bake for 20-25 minutes or until tender

MAKES 2 SERVINGS

ROASTED VEGETABLES

Works with: Intermittent Fasting | Ketogenic | Low-Carb | Paleo | Elimination | Anti-Inflammatory | Vegan | Mediterranean | Low-Calorie

Ingredients:

6-10 small carrots, yellow, purple and orange, sliced lengthwise
½ pound Brussels spouts, sliced in half
½ red onion, sliced
1-2 tablespoon extra virgin olive oil
1 teaspoon sea salt
½ teaspoon ground black pepper

Directions:

Pre-heat oven to 400 degrees. Place all ingredients on a baking tray and drizzle with extra virgin olive oil. Add salt and pepper.

Bake for 15-20 minutes or until vegetables are tender.

MAKES 2 SERVINGS

STEAMED ASPARAGUS

Works with: Intermittent Fasting | Ketogenic | Low-Carb | Paleo | Elimination | Anti-Inflammatory | Vegan | Mediterranean | Low-Calorie

Ingredients:

1 bunch asparagus

Directions:

Clean and cut asparagus. Bring 1 inch water and salt to boil in saucepan with steamer. Add asparagus, and cover, reduce heat to medium, and cook for 4-6 minutes, or until asparagus is bright green and tender.

MAKES 2 SERVINGS

STEAMED BROCCOLI

Works with: Intermittent Fasting | Ketogenic | Low-Carb | Paleo | Elimination | Anti-Inflammatory | Vegan | Mediterranean | Low-Calorie

Ingredients:

1 head broccoli

Directions:

Rinse broccoli, cut off stalk, and break into bite-size pieces. Bring 1-inch water and salt to boil in saucepan with steamer. Add broccoli, and cover, reduce heat to medium, and cook for 4-6 minutes, or until broccoli is bright green and tender.

MAKES 4 SERVINGS

DRESSINGS

GREEK VINAIGRETTE

Works with: Intermittent Fasting | Ketogenic | Low-Carb | Mediterranean | Low-Calorie

Ingredients:

¼ cup extra virgin olive oil
2 tablespoons red wine vinegar
2 tablespoons fresh oregano, chopped or 1 tablespoon dried
1 tablespoon feta, crumbled (optional*)
½ teaspoon sea salt
¼ teaspoon black pepper

Directions:

In a small jar (with lid) or bowl mix together the oil and vinegar. Add oregano, feta, salt and pepper and mix well.

MAKES APPROXIMATELY ½ CUP

Eliminate feta for paleo, raw, elimination, anti-inflammatory and vegan diets

WALNUT VINAIGRETTE

*Works with: Intermittent Fasting | Ketogenic | Low-Carb | Paleo |
Raw | Elimination | Anti-Inflammatory | Vegan | Mediterranean*

Ingredients:

¼ cup extra virgin olive oil
¼ cup walnut pieces
2 tablespoons apple cider vinegar
1 teaspoon Dijon mustard
1 clove garlic
½ teaspoon sea salt
¼ teaspoon ground black pepper

Directions:

Combine ingredients in a mini food processor or blender and blend
till smooth.

Extra dressing can be stored for 3-5 days in the refrigerator. Shake
well before using.

MAKES APPROXIMATELY ½ CUP

WHITE BALSAMIC VINAIGRETTE

Works with: Intermittent Fasting | Ketogenic | Low-Carb | Paleo | Raw | Elimination | Anti-Inflammatory | Vegan | Mediterranean | Low-Calorie

Ingredients:

2 tablespoons white balsamic vinegar
½ cup extra virgin olive oil
½ teaspoon sea salt
¼ teaspoon ground black pepper

Directions:

In a small stainless bowl, pour in the white balsamic vinegar. Slowly pour in the olive oil as you aggressively whisk until thoroughly combined. Add salt and pepper and whisk some more.

Store unused dressing in the refrigerator for 3-5 days.

MAKES ABOUT 1 CUP

SNACKS

APPLE AND ALMOND BUTTER

Works with: Intermittent Fasting | Raw | Elimination | Anti-Inflammatory | Vegan | Mediterranean

Ingredients:

1 medium apple, sliced
1 tablespoon fresh almond butter

Directions:

Slice apple and either spread almond butter on slices or dip slices into almond butter. Enjoy!

MAKES 1 SERVING

HOMEMADE TRAIL MIX

Works with: Intermittent Fasting | Raw | Elimination | Anti-Inflammatory | Vegan | Mediterranean

Ingredients:

1 tablespoon dried cherries
1 tablespoon raw pumpkin seeds
1 tablespoon sliced almonds
4 dried apricots, sliced
1 tablespoon coconut
2 figs, quartered

Directions:

In a small bowl, combine cherries, pumpkin seeds, almonds, apricots, coconut, and figs. Place in a jar or sealable bag and have ready for snacking.

MAKES 2 SERVINGS

WHITE BEAN HUMMUS AND VEGGIES

Works with: Intermittent Fasting | Elimination | Anti-Inflammatory | Vegan | Mediterranean | Low-Calorie

Ingredients:

1 garlic clove, crushed
2 tablespoons Tahini sesame seed paste
2 tablespoons freshly squeezed lime juice
1 tablespoon extra virgin olive oil
¾ teaspoon salt
1 (15 oz) can navy beans rinsed and drained
2-4 tablespoons water (use more or less, based on desired consistency)
6 baby carrots
4 celery stalks, halved
½ cucumber, sliced

Directions:

In food processor, combine garlic, tahini, lime juice, olive oil and salt. Blend for 30 seconds. Scrape mixture from sides of food processor. Add half the beans and blend for 1 minute. Scrape mixture from sides and add remaining beans. Add water for desired consistency. Serve with fresh vegetables. Cover and refrigerate any leftover hummus.

MAKES 2 SERVINGS

APPENDIX II:

DIET STACKING ONLINE CHALLENGE

TAKE THE CHALLENGE

I want you to reach your weight loss goals and I'm here to support you! If you're ready to lose weight and get healthy you can reach your goals by following the steps-by-step Diet Stacking program outlined in this book. If you want to take it one step further and get additional support and reach your goals much more easily then the Diet Stacking Online Challenge is for you. Go to DawnaStone.com/DietStacking to learn more.

With the Diet Stacking online challenge, you will have everything you need to succeed and I will personally be your guide on this incredible journey. As part of the Diet Stacking Weight Loss Challenge you will receive:

Four video tutorials

- Welcome video
- The Simple Stack explained
- The Weight Loss Stack explained
- The Extreme Stack explained

Detailed and easy-to-follow meal plans

- Simple Stack Meal Plan
- Weight Loss Stack Meal Plan
- Extreme Stack Meal Plan

Shopping lists

50+ Diet Stacking Recipes (with photos)

Frequently Asked Questions Handbook

In addition, you will receive **three downloadable guides** to help ensure your success:

- The Beginner's Guide to Diet Stacking
- Diet Stacking Success Tips
- Diet Stacking 101: The Rules

Plus, if you sign up today, you'll receive **three incredible bonuses**!

- 4 Anti-Inflammatory Recipes
- 27 Detox Water Recipes
- 10 Best Smoothies

LET'S DO IT TOGETER!

TAKE THE ONLINE DIET STACKING WEIGHT LOSS CHALLENGE!

Stacking Videos...Beginner's Guide...
Meal Plans...Shopping Lists...Diet Stacking
Rules...50+ Recipes (with photos)...Diet
Stacking Approved Diets...FAQ's...and more!

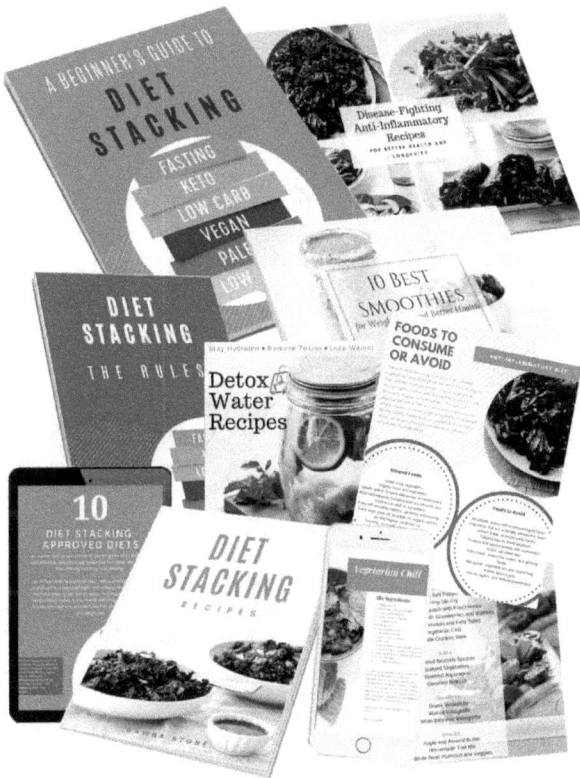

LEARN MORE AND SIGN UP AT
DAWNASTONE.COM/DIETSTACKING

APPENDIX III:

21-DAY STACKING JOURNAL

DIET STACKING JOURNAL

DAY _____

Diet Stacking Approved Diet: _____

Weight: _____

Breakfast:

Lunch:

Snack (optional):

Dinner:

Exercise:

Notes:

DIET STACKING JOURNAL

DAY _____

Diet Stacking Approved Diet: _____

Weight: _____

Breakfast:

Lunch:

Snack (optional):

Dinner:

Exercise:

Notes:

DIET STACKING JOURNAL

DAY _____

Diet Stacking Approved Diet: _____

Weight: _____

Breakfast:

Lunch:

Snack (optional):

Dinner:

Exercise:

Notes:

DIET STACKING JOURNAL

DAY _____

Diet Stacking Approved Diet: _____

Weight: _____

Breakfast:

Lunch:

Snack (optional):

Dinner:

Exercise:

Notes:

DIET STACKING JOURNAL

DAY _____

Diet Stacking Approved Diet: _____

Weight: _____

Breakfast:

Lunch:

Snack (optional):

Dinner:

Exercise:

Notes:

DIET STACKING JOURNAL

DAY _____

Diet Stacking Approved Diet: _____

Weight: _____

Breakfast:

Lunch:

Snack (optional):

Dinner:

Exercise:

Notes:

DIET STACKING JOURNAL

DAY _____

Diet Stacking Approved Diet: _____

Weight: _____

Breakfast:

Lunch:

Snack (optional):

Dinner:

Exercise:

Notes:

DIET STACKING JOURNAL

DAY _____

Diet Stacking Approved Diet: _____

Weight: _____

Breakfast:

Lunch:

Snack (optional):

Dinner:

Exercise:

Notes:

DIET STACKING JOURNAL

DAY _____

Diet Stacking Approved Diet: _____

Weight: _____

Breakfast:

Lunch:

Snack (optional):

Dinner:

Exercise:

Notes:

DIET STACKING JOURNAL

DAY _____

Diet Stacking Approved Diet: _____

Weight: _____

Breakfast:

Lunch:

Snack (optional):

Dinner:

Exercise:

Notes:

DIET STACKING JOURNAL

DAY _____

Diet Stacking Approved Diet: _____

Weight: _____

Breakfast:

Lunch:

Snack (optional):

Dinner:

Exercise:

Notes:

DIET STACKING JOURNAL

DAY _____

Diet Stacking Approved Diet: _____

Weight: _____

Breakfast:

Lunch:

Snack (optional):

Dinner:

Exercise:

Notes:

DIET STACKING JOURNAL

DAY _____

Diet Stacking Approved Diet: _____

Weight: _____

Breakfast:

Lunch:

Snack (optional):

Dinner:

Exercise:

Notes:

DIET STACKING JOURNAL

DAY _____

Diet Stacking Approved Diet: _____

Weight: _____

Breakfast:

Lunch:

Snack (optional):

Dinner:

Exercise:

Notes:

DIET STACKING JOURNAL

DAY _____

Diet Stacking Approved Diet: _____

Weight: _____

Breakfast:

Lunch:

Snack (optional):

Dinner:

Exercise:

Notes:

DIET STACKING JOURNAL

DAY _____

Diet Stacking Approved Diet: _____

Weight: _____

Breakfast:

Lunch:

Snack (optional):

Dinner:

Exercise:

Notes:

DIET STACKING JOURNAL

DAY _____

Diet Stacking Approved Diet: _____

Weight: _____

Breakfast:

Lunch:

Snack (optional):

Dinner:

Exercise:

Notes:

DIET STACKING JOURNAL

DAY _____

Diet Stacking Approved Diet: _____

Weight: _____

Breakfast:

Lunch:

Snack (optional):

Dinner:

Exercise:

Notes:

DIET STACKING JOURNAL

DAY _____

Diet Stacking Approved Diet: _____

Weight: _____

Breakfast:

Lunch:

Snack (optional):

Dinner:

Exercise:

Notes:

DIET STACKING JOURNAL

DAY _____

Diet Stacking Approved Diet: _____

Weight: _____

Breakfast:

Lunch:

Snack (optional):

Dinner:

Exercise:

Notes:

DIET STACKING JOURNAL

DAY _____

Diet Stacking Approved Diet: _____

Weight: _____

Breakfast:

Lunch:

Snack (optional):

Dinner:

Exercise:

Notes:

ENDNOTES

1   Tomiyama, A. J., Ahlstrom, B., & Mann, T. (2013). Long-term effects of dieting: Is weight loss related to health? Social and Personality Psychology Compass, 7(12), 861–877. https://doi.org/10.1111/spc3.12076

2   Centers for Disease Control. (2018). Adult obesity facts. Website. Retrieved from https://www.cdc.gov/obesity/data/adult.html

3   Foxcroft, L. (2012). *Calories and Corsets: a history of dieting over two thousand years*. Profile Books.

4   Thomas, D. M., Gonzalez, M. C., Pereira, A. Z., Redman, L. M., & Heymsfield, S. B. (2014). Time to correctly predict the amount of weight loss with dieting. *Journal of the Academy of Nutrition and Dietetics*, *114*(6), 857-861.

5   Mc Morrow, L., Ludbrook, A., Macdiarmid, J. I., & Olajide, D. (2016). Perceived barriers towards healthy eating and their association with fruit and vegetable consumption. *Journal of Public Health*, *39*(2), 330-338.

6   Nizhebetskiy, D. (2018). Expectancy Theory and how to develop people with motivation in mind. LinkedIn. Retrieved from https://www.linkedin.com/pulse/expectancy-theory-how-develop-people-motivation-mind-nizhebetskiy/

7   Watson, L. (2015). Humans have shorter attention span than goldfish, thanks to smartphones. *The Telegraph*, *15*.

8   Zaniboni, S., Truxillo, D. M., & Fraccaroli, F. (2013). Differential effects of task variety and skill variety on burnout and turnover intentions for older and younger workers. *European Journal of Work and Organizational Psychology, 22*(3), 306-317.

9   Hankey, C., Klukowska, D., & Lean, M. (2015). A Systematic Review of the Literature on Intermittent Fasting for Weight Management. *The FASEB Journal, 29*(1_supplement), 117-4.

10   Gunners, K. (2016). 10 Evidence-Based Health Benefits of Intermittent Fasting. Healthline.com. Retrieved from https://www.healthline.com/nutrition/10-health-benefits-of-intermittent-fasting

11   Hankey, 2015.

12   Mattson, M. P., Longo, V. D., & Harvie, M. (2017). Impact of intermittent fasting on health and disease processes. *Ageing research reviews, 39,* 46-58.

13   Gunners, 2016.

14   Wolver, S., Konjeti, V. R., Carbone, S., Abbate, A., & Puri, P. (2017). Successful Weight Loss with Low-carbohydrate Ketogenic Diet (LCKD) Significantly Reduced Visceral Fat and Increased Fat Free Mass in Obese. *Gastroenterology, 152*(5), S831.

15   Mawer, R. (2017). 10 Graphs That Show the Power of a Ketogenic Diet. Healthline.com. Retrieved from https://www.healthline.com/nutrition/10-graphs-power-of-ketogenic-diet#section2

16   Gibson, A. A., Seimon, R. V., Lee, C. M., Ayre, J., Franklin, J., Markovic, T. P., ... & Sainsbury, A. (2015). Do ketogenic diets really suppress appetite? A systematic review and meta-analysis. *Obesity Reviews, 16*(1), 64-76.

17   Azar, S. T., Beydoun, H. M., & Albadri, M. R. (2016). Benefits of ketogenic diet for management of type two diabetes: a review. *J Obes Eat Disord*, *2*(2).

18   Ibid.

19   Gardner, C. D., Trepanowski, J. F., Del Gobbo, L. C., Hauser, M. E., Rigdon, J., Ioannidis, J. P., ... & King, A. C. (2018). Effect of low-fat vs low-carbohydrate diet on 12-month weight loss in overweight adults and the association with genotype pattern or insulin secretion: the DIETFITS randomized clinical trial. *Jama*, *319*(7), 667-679.

20   Noakes, T. D., & Windt, J. (2017). Evidence that supports the prescription of low-carbohydrate high-fat diets: a narrative review. *Br J Sports Med*, *51*(2), 133-139.

21   Gunners, K. (2017). 23 Studies on Low-Carb and Low-Fat Diets — Time to Retire the Fad. Healthline. com. Retrieved from https://www.healthline.com/ nutrition/23-studies-on-low-carb-and-low-fat-diets#section10

22   Noakes, 2017.

23   Ibid.

24   Gunners, K. (2014). 5 Studies on The Paleo Diet – Does it Actually Work? Healthline.com. Retrieved from https://www. healthline.com/nutrition/5-studies-on-the-paleo-diet

25   Jones, Michael. (2017). Post- Dinner Satiety with the Paleolithic Diet Compared to Usual Diet. *Honors Projects*. 599. Retrieved from https://scholarworks.gvsu.edu/ honorsprojects/599

26   Gunners, 2014.

27   Masharani, U., Sherchan, P., Schloetter, M., Stratford, S., Xiao, A., Sebastian, A., ... & Frassetto, L. (2015). Metabolic and physiologic effects from consuming a hunter-gatherer (Paleolithic)-type diet in type 2 diabetes. *European journal of clinical nutrition, 69*(8), 944.

28   Frassetto, L. A., Schloetter, M., Mietus-Synder, M., Morris, R. C., & Sebastian, A. (2015). Metabolic and physiologic improvements from consuming a paleolithic, hunter-gatherer type diet (vol 69, pg 1376, 2015).

29   U.S. News and World Report. (2018). What is raw food diet? Retrieved from https://health.usnews.com/best-diet/raw-food-diet

30   Najjar, R. (2017). *Effects of a Four Week Raw, Plant-Based Diet on Anthropometric and Cardiovascular Risk Factors* (Doctoral dissertation, Texas Woman's University).

31   Raman, R. (2017). How to Do an Elimination Diet and Why. Healthline.com. Retrieved from https://www.healthline.com/nutrition/elimination-diet

32   Fox News. (2013). The new science of weight loss: Introducing the anti-inflammatory diet. Retrieved from https://www.foxnews.com/health/the-new-science-of-weight-loss-introducing-the-anti-inflammatory-diet

33   Kaluza, J., Håkansson, N., Harris, H. R., Orsini, N., Michaëlsson, K., & Wolk, A. (2019). Influence of anti-inflammatory diet and smoking on mortality and survival in men and women: two prospective cohort studies. *Journal of internal medicine.*

34   Cottam, D. R., Mattar, S. G., Barinas-Mitchell, E., Eid, G., Kuller, L., Kelley, D. E., & Schauer, P. R. (2004). The chronic inflammatory hypothesis for the morbidity associated with morbid obesity: implications and effects of weight loss. *Obesity surgery*, *14*(5), 589-600.

35   Turner-McGrievy, G., Mandes, T., & Crimarco, A. (2017). A plant-based diet for overweight and obesity prevention and treatment. *Journal of geriatric cardiology: JGC*, *14*(5), 369.

36   Olabi, A., Levitsky, D. A., Hunter, J. B., Spies, R., Rovers, A. P., & Abdouni, L. (2015). Food and mood: A nutritional and mood assessment of a 30-day vegan space diet. *Food quality and preference*, *40*, 110-115.

37   Turner-McGrievy, 2017.

38   Chertoff, J. (2016). Vegan vs. Vegetarian: The Differences and Health Facts. Healthline.com. Retrieved from https://www.healthline.com/health/food-nutrition/vegetarian-vs-vegan#1

39   Ibid.

40   Gunners, K. (2017). 5 Studies on The Mediterranean Diet - Does it Really Work? Healthline.com. Retrieved from https://www.healthline.com/nutrition/5-studies-on-the-mediterranean-diet

41   Ibid.

42   Ibid.

43   Steven, S., Hollingsworth, K. G., Al-Mrabeh, A., Avery, L., Aribisala, B., Caslake, M., & Taylor, R. (2016). Very-low-calorie diet and 6 months of weight stability in type 2 diabetes: pathophysiologic changes in responders and nonresponders. *Diabetes care*, dc151942.

44   Ibid.

45   Fung, J. (2015). Fasting: A history Part I. Intensive Dietary Management. Retrieved from https://idmprogram.com/fasting-a-history-part-i/

46   BBC News. (2012). The power of intermittent fasting. BBC News. Retrieved from https://www.bbc.com/news/health-19112549

47   PopCulture.com staff. (2018). 10 Celebrities That Swear by Intermittent Fasting. PopCulture.com. Retrieved from https://popculture.com/healthy-living/2018/08/13/10-celebrities-that-swear-by-intermittent-fasting/#2

48   Wheless, J. W. (2008). History of the ketogenic diet. *Epilepsia, 49*, 3-5.

49   Ibid.

50   Ibid.

51   Campos, M. (2018). Ketogenic diet: Is the ultimate low-carb diet good for you? Harvard Health. Retrieved from https://www.health.harvard.edu/blog/ketogenic-diet-is-the-ultimate-low-carb-diet-good-for-you-2017072712089

52   Ibid.

53   Ibid.

54   Newsmax Health. (2015). Low-Carb Diet Was Invented 225 Years Ago. Retrieved from https://www.newsmax.com/health/health-news/low-carb-diet-nutrition-fat/2015/03/19/id/631186/

55   Heffernan, C. (2014). The history of the low-carb diet. *Physical Culture Study*. Retrieved from https://physicalculturestudy.com/2014/10/04/the-history-of-the-low-carb-diet/

56   Atkins.com. (2018). Atkin's history. Retrieved from https://www.atkins.com/our-story/atkins-diet-history

57   Sima, Alexandra. (2018). Low-carb Diet–To Love or to Hate? *Romanian Journal of Diabetes Nutrition and Metabolic Diseases*, 25, 3, 233-236.

58   Ibid.

59   Ibid.

60   Cordain, L. (2012). *AARP: The paleo diet revised: Lose weight and get healthy by eating the foods you were designed to eat.* John Wiley & Sons.

61   Ibid.

62   Coelho, J. (2014). Ten famous people on the Paleo diet. LA Weekly. Retrieved from https://www.laweekly.com/restaurants/first-look-bruce-marders-rooster-is-the-cock-of-the-walk-10076026

63   Aloia, D. (2015). Uncooked Foods and How to Use Them: A History of the Raw Food Diet. New York Academy of Medicine Center for History. Retrieved from https://nyamcenterforhistory.org/2015/12/02/uncooked-foods-and-how-to-use-them-a-history-of-the-raw-food-diet/#_edn4

64   U.S. News and World Report. (2018). Raw food diet. Website. Retrieved from https://health.usnews.com/best-diet/raw-food-diet

65   Ibid.

66   Adcock, K. (2016). These 11 Celebs Follow a Raw Vegan Lifestyle & Its the Secret to Their Beauty. Voolas. Retrieved from https://voolas.com/celebs-you-didnt-know-followed-a-raw-vegan-lifestyle/

67   Centers for Disease Control. (2018). Food allergy facts. CDC.gov. Retrieved from https://www.cdc.gov/healthyschools/foodallergies/index.htm

68   Rowe, A. H., Rowe, A., & Uyeyama, K. (1954). The allergic epigastric syndrome. *Journal of Allergy and Clinical Immunology*, *25*(5), 464-471.

69   Peffer, M. (2016). The One Food Gisele Bündchen, Khloé Kardashian, and Megan Fox Don't Eat. Byrdie.com. Retrieved from https://www.byrdie.com/celebrities-that-dont-eat-dairy/slide2

70   Lewis, B. (2015). Anti-inflammatory game changers: the low-carb people in recent history. PsoriasisList.com. Retrieved from http://www.psoriasislist.com/community-famous-anti-inflammatory-people.html

71   Ibid.

72   Pasternak, H. (2016). Is Gisele Bündchen and Tom Brady's Diet for You? Celeb Trainer Harley Pasternak Investigates. People.com. Retrieved from https://people.com/food/is-gisele-bundchen-and-tom-bradys-diet-for-you-celeb-trainer-harley-pasternak-investigates/

73   Hogan, B. (2017). The Anti-Inflammatory Diet Catherine Zeta-Jones Swears By. OrganicAuthority.com. Retrieved from https://www.organicauthority.com/energetic-health/how-catherine-zeta-jones-keeps-balanced-and-looking-as-beautiful-as-ever

74   The Vegan Society. (2018). About us: History. VeganSociety.com. Retrieved from https://www.vegansociety.com/about-us/history

75   Ibid.

76   Ballard, J. (2018). 26 Celebrities You Didn't Know Were Vegan. *Good housekeeping*. Retrieved from https://www.goodhousekeeping. com/life/g5186/vegan-celebrities/?slide=2

77   Altomare, R., Cacciabaudo, F., Damiano, G., Palumbo, V. D., Gioviale, M. C., Bellavia, M., ... & Monte, A. I. L. (2013). The mediterranean diet: a history of health. *Iranian journal of public health*, *42*(5), 449.

78   Ibid.

79   Keys, A., Menotti, A., Aravanis, C., Blackburn, H., Djordevič, B. S., Buzina, R., ... & Mohaček, I. (1984). The seven countries study: 2,289 deaths in 15 years. *Preventive medicine*, *13*(2), 141-154.

80   Ibid.

81   d'Estries, M. (2016). 5 celebrities who have benefited from the Mediterranean diet. *From the Grapevine*. Retrieved from https://www.fromthegrapevine.com/ health/5-celebrities-who-have-benefited-mediterranean-diet

82   Steven, S., Hollingsworth, K. G., Al-Mrabeh, A., Avery, L., Aribisala, B., Caslake, M., & Taylor, R. (2016). Very-low-calorie diet and 6 months of weight stability in type 2 diabetes: pathophysiologic changes in responders and nonresponders. *Diabetes care*, dc151942.

83   Mosley, M. (2018). The blood sugar diet. Retrieved from https://thebloodsugardiet.com/

84   Ibid.

85   Ibid.

86   ABC News. (2012). Anne Hathaway and More Stars Who've Done Extreme Diets. Retrieved from https://abcnews.go.com/Entertainment/anne-hathaway-stars-whove-extreme-diets/story?id=16605377

87   Sifferlin, A. (2017). The Weight Loss Trap: Why Your Diet Isn't Working. Time Magazine. Retrieved from http://time.com/magazine/us/4793878/june-5th-2017-vol-189-no-21-u-s/

88   Ibid.